MINDFULNESS-BASED RELAPSE PREVENTION
FOR ADDICTIVE BEHAVIORS

Mindfulness-Based Relapse Prevention
for Addictive Behaviors

A CLINICIAN'S GUIDE

Sarah Bowen

Neha Chawla

G. Alan Marlatt

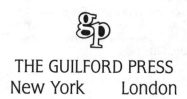

THE GUILFORD PRESS
New York   London

LIMITED PHOTOCOPY LICENSE

These materials are intended for use only by qualified professionals.

The Publisher grants to individual purchasers of this book nonassignable
permission to reproduce all materials for which photocopying permission is
specifically granted in a footnote. This license is limited to you, the individual
purchaser, for personal use or use with individual clients. This license does
not grant the right to reproduce these materials for resale, redistribution,
electronic display, or any other purposes (including but not limited to books,
pamphlets, articles, video- or audiotapes, blogs, file-sharing sites, Internet
or intranet sites, and handouts or slides for lectures, workshops, webinars,
or therapy groups, whether or not a fee is charged). Permission to reproduce
these materials for these and any other purposes must be obtained in writing
from the Permissions Department of Guilford Publications.

Library of Congress Cataloging-in-Publication Data

Bowen, Sarah.
  Mindfulness-based relapse prevention for addictive behaviors : a clinician's
guide / Sarah Bowen, Neha Chawla, G. Alan Marlatt.
       p. cm.
  Includes bibliographical references and index.
  ISBN 978-1-60623-987-2 (pbk.: alk. paper)
    1. Substance abuse—Relapse—Prevention.   2. Compulsive behavior—
Relapse—Prevention.   3. Substance abuse—Treatment.   4. Compulsive
behavior—Treatment.   5. Mindfulness-based cognitive therapy.   I. Chawla,
Neharika.   II. Marlatt, G. Alan.   III. Title.
  RC564.B68 2011
  616.89′1425—dc22
                                                                    2010037035

About the Authors

Sarah Bowen, PhD, is a research scientist and therapist in the Addictive Behaviors Research Center at the University of Washington, where she specializes in mindfulness practice for the treatment of addictive behaviors. Her research has focused specifically on mechanisms of change, including negative affect, thought suppression, and craving. She is particularly interested in the application of mindfulness-based work to dual-diagnosis populations. Dr. Bowen has co-facilitated mindfulness-based relapse prevention groups in numerous settings, including private and county treatment agencies and the VA Medical Center in Seattle. She also presents, consults, and teaches on the use of mindfulness-based treatment for substance use disorders.

Neha Chawla, PhD, is a postdoctoral fellow in the Addictive Behaviors Research Center at the University of Washington. Her research focuses on the development and evaluation of mindfulness-based treatments for substance use disorders, issues related to therapist training and dissemination, and the assessment of therapist competence. Dr. Chawla has facilitated numerous mindfulness-based relapse prevention groups in private and community treatment settings in Seattle and on the East Coast, and has co-led several therapist training workshops.

G. Alan Marlatt, PhD, is Director of the Addictive Behaviors Research Center, Professor of Psychology, and Adjunct Professor in the School of Public Health at the University of Washington. His major focus in both research and clinical work is the field of addictive behaviors. In addition to over 250 journal articles and book chapters, he has published several books in the addictions field, including *Relapse*

Prevention (1985, 2005), *Assessment of Addictive Behaviors* (1988, 2005), *Harm Reduction* (1998), and *Brief Alcohol Screening and Intervention for College Students (BASICS): A Harm Reduction Approach* (1999). Over the course of the past 30 years, Dr. Marlatt has received continuous funding for his research from a variety of agencies, including the National Institute on Alcohol Abuse and Alcoholism, the National Institute on Drug Abuse, ABMRF/The Foundation for Alcohol Research, and the Robert Wood Johnson Foundation. He is a recipient of the Jellinek Memorial Award for outstanding contributions to knowledge in the field of alcohol studies (1990), the Robert Wood Johnson Foundation's Innovators in Combating Substance Abuse Award (2001), and the Research Society on Alcoholism's Distinguished Researcher Award (2004). In 2010, he received the Association of Behavioral and Cognitive Therapy's Career/Lifetime Achievement Award.

Preface

Mindfulness-based relapse prevention (MBRP) is a program integrating mindfulness meditation practices with traditional relapse prevention (RP). Traditional RP is a cognitive-behavioral intervention designed to help prevent or manage relapse for clients following treatment for addictive behavior problems. Similarly, MBRP is designed as an outpatient aftercare program to support maintenance of treatment gains and to foster a sustainable lifestyle for individuals in recovery. In this book we present clinical strategies in the treatment of alcohol and other substance use problems. We also discuss methods for coping with urges and cravings that might be triggers for relapse across a variety of addictive behaviors. This Preface sets the stage for the material presented in this book by providing an account of how previous research and experience led to the emergence of MBRP.

Much of the present research has been informed by a quest for what has been termed the "middle way," or a balance between harmful indulgence and strict renunciation as well as between self-discipline and self-compassion. I began my career with a study evaluating electrical aversion therapy in the treatment of alcohol dependence. Aversion therapy is a punishment procedure designed to transform craving into an aversive response, marked by a desire to avoid or escape pain to prevent the urge to drink or take drugs. As we discovered, although this treatment approach may be effective in the short run, individuals in aversion therapy often have a higher relapse potential in the long run.

As our research developed, my colleagues and I found ourselves moving toward a more balanced approach. We have come a long way since, and realized that incorporating mindful skills, based on principles of self-compassion and acceptance of all experiences, including craving and urges, may be more successful than aversion approaches in lowering relapse risk. Mindfulness practice provides effective and skillful means for diligent, intentional behavior change, while emphasizing kindness and flexibility.

Addiction is considered by many individuals (including those who self-identify as "addicts") to be a moral problem deserving of punishment. In the "war on drugs," illegal drug users are put in jail to punish them for their immoral and illegal behavior, another extension of the aversion approach. Addicts are often viewed as responsible for their "bad habit" of continuing to abuse substances. They often experience considerable guilt and shame about their abuse of alcohol and other drugs, and are not likely to voluntarily seek out treatment for fear of rejection and punishment. Many of these individuals will eventually end up either forced into treatment, often as a result of a confrontational "intervention" by family members and peers, or incarcerated following a substance-related offense. These consequences only add to their stigma and shame.

My search for a middle way led me to wonder if there was another, perhaps more positive, perspective on the nature and origins of addiction. Buddhist psychology provides a promising route to recovery that offers an alternative and perhaps complementary means to overcome addictive behavior. According to the "Four Noble Truths" outlined by the Buddha, life is fraught with suffering (first Truth), and this suffering is caused by attachment or craving. This can take several forms, such as craving for sense pleasures, wanting to be someone different, or reaching for what comes next. It can also take the form of aversion or struggling against "what is" (second Truth). The good news is that there is a way out of this suffering (third Truth) provided by the "eight-fold path" (fourth Truth).

The eight-fold path provides a list of the eight desirable behaviors (or what are termed in Buddhism "right" behaviors) and associated mental states, including "right mindfulness" based on the practice of meditation. (The other steps on this path are consistent with many cognitive-behavioral treatment goals, including "right view, intention, speech, action, livelihood, effort, and concentration.") The eight-fold path and Buddhist psychology in general deal with the very issues that so often arise in the treatment of addictions and thus provide not only a foundation for our understanding of addictive behaviors, but specific interventions that address the problems that often keep recovery at bay.

But what does mindfulness specifically offer to the addictive behaviors field? As defined by Jon Kabat-Zinn (1994), mindfulness is "a way of paying attention: on purpose, in the present moment, and nonjudgmentally" (p. 4). Our focus in applying mindfulness clinically is on helping individuals with addictive behaviors "see things the way they really are" instead of focusing on the future and finding their "next fix." Buddhist psychology emphasizes acknowledging, feeling, and accepting discomfort when it arises, and understanding the experience intimately, rather than endlessly attempting to run away from it. This is a compassionate approach, emphasizing acceptance and openness rather than guilt, blame, and shame about one's behavior. Mindfulness also promotes awareness of the changing nature of things; our minds, bodies, and environments are in a constant state of change. For example, consider the smoker who cannot imagine going 45 minutes without a cigarette, but who doesn't realize that his or her seemingly overwhelming desires may attenuate if he or she can just ride them out. Mindfulness can provide a "skillful means" of coping with urges and craving that involves observing them, without being wiped out or consumed by them. Even though the smoker may feel that the urge to smoke will increase unless he or she gives in and lights up a cigarette, the smoker's urges and craving will change on their own if he or she gives them time to pass.

Additionally, mindfulness provides a state of metacognitive awareness in which one can see more of the "big picture" instead of giving into one's usual conditioned, habitual behavior. This awareness provides a greater sense of freedom and choice. As stated by Viktor Frankl (1946), "Between stimulus and response, there is a space. In that space is our power to choose our response. In our response lies our growth and freedom." Mindfulness practices increase awareness of this space and create the opportunity to respond skillfully rather than react automatically and habitually. Thus, when faced with a trigger for substance use, one can make a mindful choice that decreases the likelihood of relapse. Finally, a mindful approach can help reduce the tendency of the mind to exacerbate negative emotional states, lowering the stigma, shame, blame, and guilt commonly experienced by people who struggle with addictive behaviors.

In considering my personal journey from practicing aversion therapy to mindfulness, many paths have led me to this juncture. The first of these was my effort to discover what led people to relapse. One of my first clinical patients was a middle-aged man who was diagnosed with alcohol dependence. My clinical supervisor at Napa State Hospital, where I was doing a predoctoral internship, recommended an insight-development approach ostensibly designed to help my patient understand why he had become a problem drinker, why he should make a lifelong goal of abstinence, why he should attend Alcoholics Anonymous, and why he needed to be in an inpatient treatment program. Having worked with him to facilitate his understanding of why he should give up drinking for the rest of his life, I felt confident that his level of motivation for recovery was well established when he completed the program. On the day of his discharge, I saw him off on the Greyhound Bus headed for San Francisco, his hometown.

Less than 3 days later, he returned to Napa State, severely intoxicated, and was readmitted to the detox unit. When I asked him what had happened after his discharge, he told me that his bus made its first stop in the Tenderloin district of San Francisco, right in front of a bar that he had regularly frequented. He said he thought one of his close friends might be inside, so he walked straight from the bus into the bar. His friend was not there, but the bartender recognized him and poured him a free double-shot of whiskey as a way of welcoming him back. He described a "loss of control" over the next hour, during which he continued to drink until he passed out. A friend had him readmitted the next day. After telling me this story, he said, "Dr. Marlatt, you were very persuasive in helping me understand *why* I had become an alcoholic, and *why* I should give up drinking, and *why* abstinence was my only pathway to recovery. But you never said a damn thing about *how* I was supposed to achieve this goal!"

After this interview, I approached the Director of the Alcoholism Treatment Center at Napa and asked why, given the high relapse rates of patients treated in the program, we didn't give patients any information about how to cope with relapse. He looked at me askance and replied, "We're definitely not going to talk about relapse, because if we did that, we would be giving them permission to do so." I countered by asking why we need to have fire drills; these procedures are not designed to give people permission to set fires but to keep them safe and alive in the event of one. He replied that relapse was a sensitive issue and not to be encouraged in any way. It was at this point that I saw the moral model in action and realized it wasn't working. But what alternative could we offer? I was inspired to look more closely at what caused relapse. In addition, given that my doctoral training focused on behavior therapy, I became interested in examining a variety of behavioral interventions that might help in the development for a cognitive-behavioral program for relapse prevention.

After my internship at Napa State Hospital and a brief sojourn at the University of British Columbia, I accepted a new assistant professorship at the University of Wisconsin. I began doing clinical work with patients in the alcoholism treatment ward at Mendota State Hospital. In the late 1960s, the literature on behavior therapy approaches to treating alcoholism advocated aversion therapy more highly than most other interventions. As noted earlier, its purpose is to transform craving and urges to drink into an aversive response that deters further consumption. This is based on classical conditioning principles and is designed to elicit a conditioned response when the patient is presented with alcoholic beverages and associated drinking cues.

To further explore aversion therapy for use with addictions treatment, I received a grant to construct a small bar in the basement of the hospital in which patients from the regular month-long treatment program volunteered to be randomly assigned either to receive aversion therapy or to be in the treatment-as-usual control group. All of the patients in the study were male, most of them with long histories of alcohol dependence. For the electrical aversion procedure, each patient selected a shock level that was painful but not physically harmful. During the twice-weekly sessions in the bar (which hospital staff nicknamed "Marlatt's Bar and GRILL"), patients were presented with their favorite alcoholic beverage and asked to pick up the glass and look at and smell the drink, but not to consume any of it. At that point, a brief shock was administered to create a conditioned aversion to the alcoholic beverage (Okulitch & Marlatt, 1972).

After the patients were released, we conducted follow-up assessments at 3 months posttreatment and again a year later (15 months posttreatment). At the 3-month follow-up, patients who completed aversion treatment had higher abstinence rates and significantly lower drinking rates than those who had been in the treatment-as-usual control group. Despite these promising initial results, a year later patients in the aversion condition showed a strong rebound effect and were drinking significantly more than patients in the control condition. Not only had the aversion effects worn off over time, but the participants ended up drinking even more than patients who had been in the regular hospital program.

The literature on the short-term and long-term effects of punishment and aversive conditioning confirmed these results. Research suggested that punishment tended to result in the temporary suppression of target behaviors, but over time, in the absence of learning an alternative behavioral response, the suppressed behaviors tended to reappear. We realized we needed to teach alternative coping responses. As I thought about this process, it seemed important to assess the situation that precipitated the patient's first lapse after an initial period of abstinence. What were the triggers associated with taking the first drink? What happened on the day the patient first "fell off the wagon"? If we had more information on the precipitating circumstances, perhaps we could train the patient to acquire new and effective coping skills that might help prevent relapse.

In my study of aversion therapy, I wanted to know whether relapsed patients took their first drink in a situation that differed from that of the treatment environment (our simulated bar). Aversion treatment would have limited application if the effects were confined to the specific beverage and environment used in the initial treatment. As a result, we obtained detailed accounts of relapse episodes from patients in the follow-up interviews. Patients who relapsed were interviewed within a few days to obtain information about the initial lapse, including the physical location, presence or absence of others, any external or internal events that occurred prior to the lapse, and any emotions or feelings that occurred. Descriptions of the relapse episodes were coded and assigned to operationally defined categories.

Most of the relapse episodes could be assigned to surprisingly few categories. The first two areas, accounting for more than half of the cases, involved an interpersonal encounter. Almost one-third of the situations involved an episode in which the patient was frustrated in some goal-directed activity and reported feelings of anger. Rather than expressing their anger constructively, patients ended up having a drink. The second category involved social influences, with patients reporting an inability to resist direct or indirect social pressure to engage in drinking. The other categories could be described as intrapersonal, including giving in to urges or cravings often elicited by environmental stimuli (as was the case with my patient from Napa State Hospital who gave in to the urge to drink once he entered a bar setting). In subsequent studies, we found similar patterns of high-risk situations associated with relapse episodes for other addictive behaviors, including cigarette smoking and heroin use. In all, there seemed to be a common thread running through these situations that made them potential triggers for relapse: the need to "self-medicate" when the individual experienced strong negative emotional states, including anger, anxiety, depression, and interpersonal conflict.

In efforts to identify high-risk situations, we learned that although there may be a variety of underlying mediating factors involved, it is the individual's own subjective perception of "risk" that is most important. As such, a high-risk situation is defined broadly as any situation that poses a threat to one's sense of perceived control (self-efficacy) and increases the risk of potential relapse. To the extent that heavy drinking, smoking, or other substance use occurred (prior to one's commitment to abstinence) in similar situations, most users will have developed strong positive expectancies (craving) about using the drug as a coping strategy. Users come to believe they cannot cope with certain stressful situations, such as feeling angry, socializing with substance-using peers, or facing the threat of negative evaluation, unless they are able to lean on the addictive behavior as a crutch.

The most salient factor that serves to decrease the risk of relapse in an otherwise high-risk situation, and which is at the core of the RP model, is access to an alternative coping response. If the individual has acquired new ways of coping with stressful situations, we hypothesized that self-efficacy would be strengthened and the probability of relapse would decrease. RP focuses on identifying high-risk situations and teaching coping skills so as to increase self-efficacy and decrease the likelihood of relapse. After the publication of *Relapse Prevention* (Marlatt & Gordon, 1985), a variety of treatment outcome studies were completed evaluating the clinical effectiveness of RP, many of which have been summarized in the second edition (Marlatt & Donovan, 2005). The results overall show that although RP does not result in higher abstinence rates following treatment, it does significantly reduce the frequency and intensity of relapse episodes, helping people get "back on track" more quickly if they do fall off the wagon.

Over the past quarter century, we have attempted to include strong and easily adopted coping skills in our RP program. Of course, one of the most potent and readily accessible coping mechanisms we had at our disposal is mindfulness meditation. In the first edition of *Relapse Prevention*, the chapter on "Lifestyle Modification" included meditation as a cognitive coping strategy that might help provide balance for individuals at risk for relapse related to a stressful lifestyle:

> One of the most significant effects of regular meditation practice is the development of mindfulness—the capacity to observe the ongoing process of experience without at the same time becoming "attached" or identifying with the content of each thought, feeling, or image. Mindfulness is a particularly effective cognitive skill for the practice of RP. If clients can acquire this ability through the regular practice of meditation, they may be able to "detach" themselves from the lure of urges, cravings, or cognitive rationalizations that may otherwise lead to a lapse. (Marlatt & Gordon, 1985, p. 319)

My own interest in meditation began in the early 1970s, after I moved to the University of Washington in Seattle. I was experiencing the typical stress associated with the "publish or perish" demands of academic life, and my blood pressure became elevated. My physician suggested meditation as a way to relax. I became defensive, explaining that as a behavior therapist, I had no interest in participating in "Eastern" practices associated with Hinduism or Buddhism. He handed me an article showing that the regular practice of transcendental meditation (TM) lowered the diastolic blood pressure of patients being treated for hypertension. "Since you're a researcher," he said, "I thought you would be impressed with these results." He advised me to sign up for TM and give it a try for 3 months, telling me that if it did not bring my blood pressure down, he would recommend medication. "You can measure your blood pressure on a daily basis and make a graph of the results—either it will work or not, so that's the purpose of your personal research study." I agreed and signed up for TM training.

TM is known as a "concentrative meditation" technique in which the meditator focuses on a single word (a unique mantra given to each new student by the TM instructor). The instructions were to sit quietly with eyes closed for two 20-minute periods each day, repeating the mantra with each inbreath and outbreath. When distracted by other thoughts or images, I was told to gently return the attention to the mantra and to continue to sit quietly.

After considerable initial skepticism, once I began the practice, I found it to be very relaxing. I sat in the morning before going to work and again after work in the late afternoon. To my delight, my diastolic blood pressure showed a significant drop after the first 2 weeks of daily practice. My physician was also pleased and encouraged me to continue practicing TM on a long-term basis. He also recommended the book *The Relaxation Response* by physician Herbert Benson (1975). Benson included a basic meditation practice to enhance muscle relaxation and reduce tension. Clearly there was medical evidence supporting the benefits of meditation as a tension-reduction practice. Given that both ongoing addictive behavior and risk for relapse go up as tension and stress increase, both at the physiological and psychological levels, it seemed clear that meditation could be a helpful coping skill in addiction treatment.

As a result of personal and professional experience in the meditation field, my colleagues and I decided to do some outcome research to see how the practice of meditation, relaxation training, and exercise might affect the drinking behavior of male heavy social drinkers. We selected heavy drinkers rather than alcohol-dependent patients as our subjects because we wanted to determine if their daily practice (of meditation, muscle relaxation, or exercise, depending on their random assignment to condition) would affect the amount of alcohol they consumed. We did not include alcohol-dependent drinkers because treatment usually requires abstinence as the only acceptable goal. The results showed that all three of the daily practices had a significant impact on reducing drinking rates compared to the control group during the 16-week intervention period. On average, consumption rates dropped 50% from the preintervention drinking rates (Marlatt & Marques, 1977; Marlatt, Pagano, Rose, & Marques, 1984). In addition, participants continued to practice on their own volition during the follow-up period: 62% of the aerobic exercise group (running practice) and 57% of the subjects in the meditation group continued practicing their techniques regularly.

My interest in TM was limited to the extent that there was little theoretical literature showing how TM worked in terms of changing cognitive functioning and personal stress levels. Starting in the early 1980s, my interest in meditation evolved to include the study of Buddhist psychology (Marlatt, 2002). The Buddhist literature seemed parallel in many ways to cognitive-behavioral therapy, and I began doing meditation retreats with a variety of Buddhist teachers, including S. N. Goenka, the renowned teacher of *vipassana* (a Sanskrit term meaning "seeing things as they really are"). At the end of one 10-day retreat, I asked him about the Buddhist definition of addiction. After explaining that most experts in the United States defined addiction as a "disease of the brain," I posed the question "How does Buddhism define addiction?" He replied, "Yes, addiction is a disease—it's a disease of the *mind*." At that point, I realized that mindfulness meditation could be helpful for people with addictive behavior in terms of coping with urges and craving, whether they are pursuing a goal of moderation or abstinence.

Several years later, I received a call from a psychologist at a minimum-security jail in Seattle, regarding a 10-day meditation retreat based on Goenka's teachings for inmates at the facility who were willing to participate. Starting with the first course in 1997, the jail continued to offer 10-day vipassana courses for inmates who volunteered to participate. As is traditional in these courses, they were held in silence, except for meditation instructions from the teachers, questions from the participants, and a daily "dharma talk" to explain the Buddhist principles of mindfulness meditation.

The psychologist who called me said that a review of the prison records showed that inmates who took the vipassana retreat showed a significant reduction in recidivism, compared to inmates who did not take the course. She asked if I would be interested in conducting a clinical outcome study to evaluate the effects of the vipassana course, with a focus on alcohol and drug use and associated risk of recidivism. We obtained a research grant from the Robert Wood Johnson Foundation to follow up with inmates who participated in the retreat and compared their outcomes with those who chose not to take the course. Results obtained 3 months following participants' release from jail showed statistically significant reductions in alcohol (and alcohol-related harm), cocaine, and marijuana use, and improved psychiatric symptoms and enhanced optimism, compared to the control group (Bowen et al., 2006).

How could we extend this experience to a broader treatment approach? Although attending a 10-day vipassana retreat can have beneficial effects for people with both mental health and addictive behavior problems, we knew that many individuals would find attending a silent retreat of this length to be too challenging. Also we knew some might object to participating in a course based on Buddhist teachings. These issues have been addressed in the development of mindfulness treatment programs for other disorders, including chronic pain and distress (mindfulness-based stress reduction [MBSR], originally developed over 30 years ago by Jon Kabat-Zinn at the University of Massachusetts Medical School; Kabat-Zinn, 1990) and depressive relapse (mindfulness-based cognitive therapy [MBCT], developed by Zindel Segal at the University of Toronto; Segal, Williams, & Teasdale, 2002). Both the MBSR and MBCT programs are conducted in a group therapy format and consist of eight weekly outpatient sessions. Both programs train patients in secular mindfulness meditation practices and metacognitive coping skills that help them manage painful physical sensations and associated anxiety (MBSR) or triggers that might precipitate a relapse into depression following initial treatment (MBCT). Both MBSR and MBCT have been found to be effective in a series of treatment outcome studies (e.g., Kabat-Zinn et al., 1992; Roth & Creaser, 1997; Teasdale et al., 2000).

Based on the structure and format of both MBSR and MBCT, we decided to develop a parallel program for the treatment of addictive behavior, MBRP, originally described by Witkiewitz, Marlatt, and Walker (2005). As outlined in this treatment guide, MBRP consists of eight weekly sessions conducted in a group therapy format integrating cognitive-behavioral RP skills with mindfulness practices. The purpose of these practices is to increase awareness of triggers and habitual reactions, to develop a new relationship with these experiences, and to learn concrete skills to use in high-risk situations.

In stark contrast to aversion therapy, which is designed to punish one's craving responses, mindfulness practice can foster exploration and acceptance of craving and urges. Instead of giving in to the desire for immediate gratification, mindfulness practice provides an opportunity to observe the cresting of the craving wave without getting "wiped out" by it. As one of my clients observed, the words *addiction* and *dictation* have the same Latin stem: *dicere* ("to impose or give orders with or as with authority"). She observed, "I still think I want to drink a lot when I get depressed, but since I finished the meditation course, I no longer have to be dictated to by my thoughts. I accept them and let them pass." By moving from aversion to acceptance as a means of coping with craving, recovery is facilitated on the basis of a new compassionate approach, which is what we hope to offer in the MBRP program.

G. Alan Marlatt

Acknowledgments

We extend tremendous gratitude to the following individuals for their substantial contributions to the development of the mindfulness-based relapse prevention (MBRP) program and guidebook. These teachers, colleagues, and friends have offered their collaboration, support, talent, and wisdom to the creation of this program.

The structure and content of MBRP are largely inspired by and based on the work of Jon Kabat-Zinn and colleagues at the Center for Mindfulness in Medicine, Health Care, and Society at the University of Massachusetts Medical School and the seminal work of Kabat-Zinn's mindfulness-based stress reduction program, as described in his book *Full Catastrophe Living* (1990). Additionally, several exercises are derived or adapted from the work of Zindel Segal, Mark Williams, and John Teasdale in *Mindfulness-Based Cognitive Therapy for Depression* (2002).

We have been extraordinarily fortunate to have had consultation and feedback from Jon Kabat-Zinn, Zindel Segal, Roger Nolan, Judson Brewer, Lisa Dale-Miller, Kevin Griffin, and Jhampa Shaneman. For their generous contribution of time and expertise as supervisors for our clinical trial, we are grateful to Judith Gordon, Madelon Bolling, Sandra Coffman, Anil Coumar, and Steven Vannoy. For their roles in the development of this program, we thank Katie Witkiewitz, Mary Larimer, Brian Ostafin, Joel Grow, Sharon Hsu, Seema Clifasefi, Susan Collins, Scott Hunt, George Parks, Anne Douglass, and Michelle Garner. For her editorial support, we thank Kitty Moore. For their unconditional support and inspiration, and for the daily opportunities for practice, we would like to thank our families, partners, and friends. For their seemingly endless wisdom and compassionate hearts, we are deeply grateful to the meditation teachers whose offerings have inspired us and deepened our own experience and understanding of the practice. Finally, for their faith, commitment, and practice, we are immensely grateful to all of the participants in our MBRP groups.

The Addictive Behaviors Research Center's Mindfulness-Based Relapse Prevention Treatment Development Project was funded by National Institute on Drug Abuse Grant No. 1 R21 DA019562-01A1, G. Alan Marlatt, PhD, Principal Investigator.

Contents

Introduction

THE MINDFULNESS-BASED RELAPSE PREVENTION (MBRP) program is as an aftercare program integrating cognitive-behavioral relapse prevention skills and mindfulness meditation practice, intended for individuals who have completed initial treatment for substance use disorders. In our experience, this program is best suited to individuals who have completed inpatient or outpatient treatment, are motivated to maintain treatment goals, and are willing to make lifestyle changes that support their well-being and recovery.

We suspect that clinicians drawn to this treatment program have significant interest in or experience with both mindfulness practice and the treatment of substance use disorders. Perhaps, similar to several of your clients, you are seeking an alternative approach or a fresh perspective to understanding and addressing substance abuse and relapse. Maybe you are seeking another means of helping your clients find freedom from the destructive cycle of these or other harmful behaviors. It is a similar search that led us to the development of MBRP.

The MBRP program is designed to bring practices of mindful awareness to individuals suffering from the addictive trappings of the mind. The practices in this program are intended to foster increased awareness of triggers, habitual patterns, and "automatic" reactions that seem to control many of our lives. These practices cultivate the ability to pause, observe present experience, and bring awareness to the range of choices before each of us in every moment. Ultimately, we are working toward freedom from deeply engrained and often catastrophic habitual patterns of thought and behavior.

The MBRP program represents a culmination of our combined experiences with treating substance use disorders. It also represents our personal journeys with meditation practice and the desire to offer to others what has been so valuable in our own lives, with the hope that it may alleviate some of their suffering. It is also through the inspiration and support of those who have pioneered mindfulness-based programs that this program has come to fruition. These individuals have paved the way for integrating these rich practices and traditions into Western science, psychology, and medicine.

We cannot overemphasize the importance of personal meditation practice as the basis for training and preparation. Although MBRP is informed by principles of cognitive and behavioral psychology, mindfulness practice is what differentiates this program from many other substance abuse treatments. Our hope is that, in the tradition of mindfulness-based stress reduction and mindfulness-based cognitive therapy, this program will remain grounded in mindfulness meditation. Familiarity and experience with cognitive therapy, facilitation of groups, and work with addictions is desirable but perhaps secondary to a foundation of personal mindfulness practice. It is their own practice that allows MBRP facilitators to model the attitudes and behaviors that they are inviting participants to cultivate and that are at the heart of the program. In our experience, there are simply no shortcuts; it is only through personal practice, and the experience of the challenges and insights that come with it, that we as facilitators can truly begin to embody the qualities MBRP is intended to foster.

For those who may be new to mindfulness practice, we strongly encourage personal exploration of mindfulness meditation before embarking upon delivery of this treatment. As a starting point, you might explore the list of meditation resources included in the final session of the program. In addition to the books and audio recordings listed there, we highly recommend direct instruction from an experienced teacher and participation in at least one intensive meditation retreat. These retreats are offered at several centers across the country, and those that offer training in insight, or vipassana meditation, are most consistent with the practices included in this program.

Part I of this book lays out the background and foundation for the development of MBRP and offers a discussion of our experience with and recommendations for training in and conducting the treatment. This includes examples of challenges encountered, lessons learned, and issues requiring further consideration. We also offer a brief overview of the initial research evaluating the efficacy of MBRP.

The remainder of this book is designed to guide readers through each of the eight sessions of the program. These chapters provide a detailed discussion of the themes and practices included in each session, along with a description of common experiences encountered by MBRP participants and possible issues that may arise. They also list materials needed, provide a structure and outline, and include worksheets, handouts, and scripted examples of the guided meditations. The first three sessions focus on practicing mindful awareness and integrating mindfulness practices into daily life. The next three sessions emphasize acceptance of present experience and application of mindfulness practices to relapse prevention, and the final two sessions expand to include issues of self-care, support networks, and lifestyle balance. Each session is designed to build on the previous one, and sessions are intended to be practiced in the order in which we describe them here. The structure offered in this program, in combination with the facilitator's personal daily mindfulness practice, is designed to offer clients new perspectives and skills to guide them not only in the day-to-day challenges of recovery but also in the moment-to-moment awareness, compassion, and freedom that mindfulness practice can bring.

PART I

Conducting Mindfulness-Based Relapse Prevention

From the outset we envisioned MBRP as an integration of standard cognitive-behavioral-based relapse prevention treatment with mindfulness meditation practices. Thus, the MBRP curriculum includes identification of personal triggers and situations in which participants are particularly vulnerable, along with practical skills to use in such times. Alongside these skills, participants learn mindfulness practices that foster a heightened awareness of and shift in one's relationship to all experiences, both internal (emotions, thoughts, sensations) and external (environmental cues), promoting a greater sense of choice, compassion, and freedom.

The program is informed by mindfulness-based stress reduction (MBSR; Kabat-Zinn, 1990), mindfulness-based cognitive therapy (MBCT; Segal, Williams, & Teasdale, 2002) and Daley and Marlatt's (2006) relapse prevention protocol. After numerous adjustments in content, structure, and style, we have arrived at a program that is increasingly inspired by and attuned to the experiences and needs of MBRP participants. MBRP continues to develop and will always be a work in progress, evolving with every new group of participants. So, although we offer a description of the MBRP course as it currently stands, it is our hope that the growing MBRP community will continue to develop it into an increasingly effective program.

In the following pages, we briefly describe our experiences with facilitating MBRP, discussing several challenges encountered and lessons learned along the way. We offer our own experience and ideas regarding selecting and training

MBRP facilitators, conducting MBRP groups, and navigating a number of logistical, theoretical, and clinical issues that may arise. Just as we have benefited immensely from the experience and advice of our MBSR and MBCT mentors, it is our hope that our experiences might be useful to those embarking upon a similar journey.

FACILITATING MBRP GROUPS

Style and Structure

The MBRP program offers a structured protocol with session-by-session agendas containing practices and worksheets integrating principles from both cognitive-behavioral therapy (CBT) and traditional mindfulness teachings. Creativity and a shared curiosity, however, are what bring the program to life. Because teachers of mindfulness meditation encourage investigation and trust of one's own experience, the core principles of MBRP are elicited from participants whenever possible and are explored through experiential practices and inquiry. This encourages participants to see their own habits of mind and patterns of behavior and to discover what is true from observation of their own experience.

Inquiry

Both the style and the structure of groups are intended to reflect an emphasis on direct experience. Sessions typically begin with experiential exercises, followed by a period of brief discussion or "inquiry" (Segal et al., 2002). The intention is to keep these discussions centered on present experience and at key points to relate that experience to relapse, recovery, craving, or lifestyle factors. Keeping inquiry focused on direct experience reflects a central intention of these mindfulness practices: to notice what is actually arising in the moment rather than getting lost in interpretations and stories. However, participants are often accustomed to telling stories *about* their experience. Facilitators, too, are often in the habit of working with content or offering potential solutions. The process here is different. It requires facilitators to continually redirect each interaction to a description of the immediate experience in the present moment (i.e., sensations in the body, thoughts, or emotions) versus the interpretation, analysis, or story about the experience. When a participant begins discussing a story, concept, or evaluating his or her experience, just as in meditation practice itself, facilitators encourage "letting go and beginning again" by redirecting the participant to the experience in the present moment. The inquiry process itself thus becomes an example of the mind's tendency to veer off into thoughts and stories and another practice in bringing focus back to present experience.

As illustrated in Figure I.1 (adapted from MBCT), the inquiry process centers on differentiating between direct experience (often sensation or emotion) and proliferations or reactions to experience (stories, judgments). The observation of direct experience is the primary intention, and repeated discernment between the initial experience and reactions to it can be helpful in recognizing when our attention has been pulled away. These reactions or "additions" might be physical (such as tension or resistance), cognitive (such as thoughts or stories), or emotional (such as frustration or yearning) and may trigger further reactions. For example, there may be a primary experience, such as an intense physical sensation, followed by a thought about that experience, such as "I can't do this" and then an emotional reaction to the thought, such as a feeling of defeat. This proliferation might continue with another thought, such as "I knew I shouldn't have come to this group."

The inquiry process helps participants distinguish between an initial experience (e.g., physical sensation) and the thoughts or reactions that might follow by encouraging them to repeatedly return their focus to what is actually occurring in the moment. With practice, participants learn to recognize when they are caught in stories or proliferations, and realize that they have the choice to pause and return to present experience. Practicing this process of recognition and returning to the present plants seeds of awareness and nonreactivity, thereby alleviating some of the undue suffering our minds often cause.

The inquiry process may also highlight ways in which the experiences arising in meditation (both the direct experiences and our reactions to it) are familiar or unfamiliar. For example, a facilitator may inquire, "How is this similar or different from what your mind usually does?" or "Have you noticed this about your mind before?" Facilitators may also ask how this experience is related to participants' lives (e.g., "How might what you just experienced be related to substance use or to relapse?"). This link between what is being experienced in the meditation and habitual patterns and behaviors may not be explicit in every interaction but is crucial to the overall purpose of the program.

Finally, inquiry is intended to be an exploration of the shared tendencies of the mind rather than of any one individual's story. As one begins to see the mind's habits more clearly, the patterns can sometimes feel very "personal" or unique to an individual, leading to frustration or a sense of being flawed. Highlighting that this is just how minds are, rather than an indication that there is "something wrong with you," can be helpful in cultivating compassion as we begin to get to know our minds a little more intimately. A facilitator might ask, "Does anyone else experience this?" or "Isn't it interesting what the mind does?" to reaffirm that these experiences are universal rather than unique to any one individual. Figure I.1 illustrates this tendency of the mind and how inquiry brings awareness to these processes.

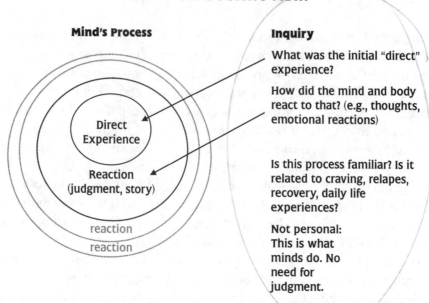

FIGURE I.1. Inquiry process. Adapted with permission from Zindel V. Segal (personal communication, March 8, 2010).

Home Practice

Home practice is assigned each week, and each session includes a review of the previous week's practices. There is a balance between encouraging and emphasizing the importance of daily practice while not inspiring self-blame and judgment. Discussing practice-related struggles with lightness, compassion, and curiosity is essential; struggles with daily mindfulness practice do not indicate another failed attempt at change, but rather represent another opportunity to observe the tendencies of the mind. Approaching these discussions functionally, nonjudgmentally, and with a sense of curiosity can help normalize common challenges, encouraging participants to view these, too, as part of practice rather than as a problem or failure. Facilitators might model this by asking, "Is anyone experiencing difficulty with practice? What thoughts or feelings do you notice when you realize you haven't practiced?"

In an effort to encourage participants to practice, facilitators may have an urge to "sell" them on the merits of meditation. Such attempts at persuasion often result in skepticism, guilt, or resistance on the part of participants. As an alternative, gently guided discussions with open-ended questions (e.g., "How do you think these practices might be helpful for relapse prevention?" or "What might help you to practice more regularly?") seem to allow group members to generate their own reasons and motivations for practice, promoting increased engagement and decreased resistance. This style of discussion seems to be the most effective approach, engendering a more cooperative, client-centered environment.

Co-Facilitation

Support from a co-facilitator can be an invaluable asset in navigating the dynamics and challenges of MBRP facilitation. It is regrettably easy to revert to habitual styles or to slip into "teaching" or "instructing" rather than eliciting themes from the group. A co-facilitator can provide a reminder or offer a different approach or perspective. Especially in the beginning stages, co-facilitators learn from one another, offering two voices and styles, keeping each other adherent to the stance and core themes of the sessions, providing support, and balancing each other's skills, perspectives, and experiences.

FACILITATORS: SELECTION, TRAINING, AND PERSONAL PRACTICE

Who Are the MBRP Facilitators?

To adequately guide the different aspects of the MBRP program, it is valuable for facilitators to have experience with substance abuse treatment and group facilitation. However, as we mentioned in the Introduction, perhaps most important is an understanding of and experience with mindfulness practice. A primary concern in developing MBRP and training facilitators has been differentiating the program from standard CBT-based relapse prevention. We were wary of creating a CBT-based treatment with the simple addition of mindfulness exercises. Instead, our intention was to create a program grounded in mindfulness practice, with relapse prevention skills presented and practiced in a way that was consistent with a mindfulness approach. Throughout the inception, training, and facilitation of groups, we have kept facilitators' mindfulness practice at the core of the treatment. We believe this is what makes the program a unique offering to the treatment community. We provide more in-depth discussion of the role of the facilitator's personal practice later (see The Importance of Personal Practice section).

Training

As with the facilitation of MBRP, we intend MBRP training to reflect the present-centered, nonjudgmental, and accepting qualities cultivated by mindfulness practice itself. The aim is to meet whatever arises—among trainees and clients alike—with curiosity, equanimity, and compassion and with an experiential, present-centered focus. We have found this to be effective not only in creating a space that supports exploration and growth but also in allowing a playful, open approach that brings both warmth and flexibility to the program.

The background and basic theory of relapse prevention, mindfulness meditation, and the blending of these practices are important pieces of the training of MBRP facilitators; however, the central focus is on experiential learning. Training can take a number of forms. For example, many facilitators have participated in 3-day workshops in which the theory and rationale are presented on the first evening, followed by 2 full days of guidance through the eight sessions of MBRP, with as many of the exercises and practices conducted in "real time" as possible. Following this initial intensive training, facilitators meet weekly for 2 months to practice leading sessions with one another, with input and supervision from the trainers. Similar to the MBRP treatment protocol, the practices and exercises precede discussions, with a significant part of each session spent on the meditations and exercises themselves. The intention is to keep the ideas and discussions simple, elaborating only in ways that would facilitate and enhance the practice itself. Trainees share questions and experiences regarding their own practice, including frustrations and barriers, such as making time in their busy schedules, the persistent wandering of the mind, self-doubt, restlessness, and sleepiness. These challenges are common to both facilitators and participants and are thus helpful to work with firsthand.

Subsequent trainings have involved a 5-day residential retreat-style format, allowing a deeper and richer experience of the program. Inspired by the MBCT training model, the format encourages trainees and facilitators to temporarily set aside the demands of their daily lives and immerse themselves in practicing together for these 5 days. The initial 2 days are spent guiding trainees through the exercises and practices of MBRP. The third day focuses on silent practice, followed by the opportunity for trainees to facilitate exercises in smaller groups, with feedback offered by both trainers and fellow trainees.

Finally, following these workshops, opportunities for trainees to observe a full 8-week session guided by experienced MBRP facilitators will further enrich the training experience, and we strongly recommend it whenever possible.

Although these formats may not always be feasible, it is highly recommended that facilitators participate in experiential training and have a background of practice before guiding MBRP. This book provides an outline for the program, but is in no way able to offer the level of understanding that comes from direct experience, observation of other facilitators, and supervision.

The Importance of Personal Practice

As we discussed, perhaps the most crucial factor in facilitating MBRP is the facilitators' personal practice of mindfulness meditation. Supporting others in the practice comes from one's own lived experience and history of having encountered similar struggles; it cannot come from simply "understanding" a treatment manual or attending a brief workshop.

Often therapists will attempt to start a meditation practice at the beginning of MBRP facilitator training. As any practitioner knows, however, consistent practice is a challenge and often takes months or even years to establish. Despite best intentions, facilitators newer to meditation often struggle with schedule constraints (i.e., allotting time for regular practice), expectations and misconceptions about mindfulness, and issues of discomfort, doubt, and self-judgment. Although these challenges are commonly experienced along the meditative journey, for practitioners who do not have the experience of an intensive retreat or support from a teacher or community, these experiences can be discouraging and difficult to navigate. We thus suggest that those who are new to this practice begin by referring to the books and meditation recordings listed in Session 8 of the program and participate in at least one 7-day or longer residential retreat in the insight meditation, or vipassana, tradition. Through practice, one discovers a different way of relating to experience that, in our observation, is in itself potentially transformative.

Given the internal nature of the meditative process, it is often difficult even for experienced facilitators to assess an individual's experience and understanding of these practices. For those with a limited understanding of the nuances of practice, this may result in a restricted ability to respond skillfully to questions, doubts, and misconceptions raised by participants. For example, one of the most common concerns that arise in the first few sessions is the expectation that the practice is supposed to bring feelings of calm and peace, and that one is "doing it wrong" or it is "not working" if he or she finds instead that the mind is distracted by thoughts, emotions, or challenging physical experiences. Facilitators with a strong personal practice may respond to such comments by drawing on their own experience for guidance, and they may be able to anticipate and explore challenges, even when participants are unable to articulate these issues themselves. As the following example illustrates, these facilitators often pick up on subtleties that are based on personal experience. (This and all subsequent dialogue was excerpted from MBRP sessions and edited for anonymity and clarity).

PARTICIPANT: I practiced with the CD you gave us every day, but I was only able to do it for about 10 minutes each time.

[At this point, a facilitator might validate the participant for practicing each day. Those with awareness of and familiarity with their own reactions during meditation may take the additional step of inquiring about what may have occurred for the participant at the end of the 10 minutes.]

FACILITATOR: So you were able to commit to practicing with the CD each day; it isn't easy to make space for something new like that in your life. I am curious what you noticed about your experience before you turned the CD off.

PARTICIPANT: I just wanted to get up and do other things.

FACILITATOR: Was there restlessness? [Redirects to the first step in the inquiry process: awareness of the immediate physical, emotional, or cognitive experience.]

PARTICIPANT: Yeah, exactly.

FACILITATOR: What does restlessness feel like to you?

PARTICIPANT: It was just a fidgety feeling, like it was hard to sit still and focus on the breath and the voice on the CD.

FACILITATOR: Any particular place in your body where you sensed that? [Continues to explore the immediate experience.]

PARTICIPANT: In my hands definitely, and sort of all over.

FACILITATOR: Hmm. What was the sensation in your hands, if you remember?

PARTICIPANT: They were sort of tingling and twitchy.

FACILITATOR: And do you remember your reaction to being restless? Were there any thoughts about it? [Inquires about reactions to immediate experience.]

PARTICIPANT: Yeah, kind of. I felt a little ashamed that I couldn't sit for more than 10 minutes.

FACILITATOR: Okay, you noticed some shame. What about thoughts? Any thoughts that you remember? [Distinguishes thoughts and emotions]

PARTICIPANT: I guess the thought that I couldn't do it anymore, that I had to get up.

FACILITATOR: Okay, feelings of restlessness in the hands and elsewhere in the body, an urge to get up and do things, and maybe a thought like "I can't do this. I have to get up." Seems like you also noticed some shame. [Highlights physical, emotional, and cognitive reactions.]

PARTICIPANT: Yeah, I felt like I should be able to sit for longer than 10 minutes.

FACILITATOR: So a thought, "I should be able to sit longer"? [Differentiates between thoughts and feeling]

PARTICIPANT: Yeah, that was all happening.

FACILITATOR: What would it be like to just notice that experience, in the same way that we have been noticing the breath, to bring the same attention and curiosity to it, as just another experience occurring in the moment? Noticing what restlessness really feels like and noticing your reaction to it. And maybe seeing if you can soften a little, just allowing it to be there and just observing it, even for a moment. And then you may make the choice to get up or not.

In this dialogue, the facilitator is encouraging awareness of the physical, emotional, and cognitive components of experience and highlighting awareness of urges that arise. She helps the participant recognize the initial experience and the several reactions that followed. She is also modeling the curiosity, openness, and nonjudgmental stance that the participant is being asked to take toward whatever arises, both during and in relation to the meditation practice. This can be validating for the participant and may help deepen the understanding of the practice, expanding it from what occurs during formal meditation to mindfulness of *all* experience. Notice, too, that she does not shift into problem solving (e.g., suggestions for how the participant might practice for longer periods of time).

Without the personal experience of having navigated one's own internal world in this way, facilitators might not respond with the same level of awareness, curiosity, and acceptance. Facilitators newer to meditation may default to what they perceive as the "right" or logical response to inquiries, subtle messages about doing it "right," or missing the misperceptions about practice that often arise. This may result in missed opportunities for deeper understanding or experience among participants.

Also challenging for facilitators new to practice is the guiding of the meditation exercises. Facilitators are strongly encouraged to guide the meditations spontaneously and from their own experience as they lead rather than reading the meditation instructions or attempting to induce a specific state by adopting a certain "meditation voice." Facilitators with extensive experience with meditation practice are typically more at ease with guiding exercises, based on their own genuine experience in the present moment. This not only brings the practice to life for both participants and facilitators but also shifts the role of the facilitator from "teacher" to someone engaging in the practice alongside the participants, enhancing the collaborative feel and alliance of the groups. As stated by Kabat-Zinn (2003), "Without the foundation of personal practice and the embodying of what it is one is teaching, attempts at mindfulness-based interventions run the risk of becoming caricatures of mindfulness, missing the radical, transformational essence."

MBRP AND 12-STEP APPROACHES

Conducting MBRP groups in the context of 12-step-oriented programs, or with participants engaged in 12-step recovery, may offer some challenges. MBRP is not in conflict with the 12-step philosophy; in fact, there are several areas of overlap, including an emphasis on acceptance, letting go of personal control, and the value of prayer and meditation (see Griffin, 2004, for an in-depth discussion of these issues). However, there are points of divergence. For example, the philosophical underpinnings of Alcoholics Anonymous (AA), Narcotics Anonymous (NA), and other 12-step approaches are a combination of the disease and spiritual models of addiction, which view substance abuse and dependence as chronic, progressive diseases of the brain (Spicer, 1993). Affected individuals are often encouraged to accept the label of "addict" or "alcoholic" and to admit "powerlessness" over their disease. They are encouraged to enlist the support of a higher power to aid them in their recovery. In contrast, the MBRP approach discourages the use of and identification with labels, positive or negative, encouraging instead an ongoing observation and acceptance of experience without ascribing value. Additionally, MBRP incorporates elements of cognitive-behavioral relapse prevention, which focus on empowering the individual through improving coping skills, exploring cognitive and behavioral antecedents of substance use, and increasing self-efficacy (Marlatt & Gordon, 1985). These practices, taken together, are intended to foster a sense of choice and agency, such that one's actions are arising from greater self-awareness, acceptance, and compassion.

Perhaps the most fundamental difference between the 12-step model and MBRP lies in their approaches to abstinence. Commitment to abstinence goals is a requirement for participation in AA and NA, whereas in MBRP, although abstinence is typically viewed as an ideal goal, it is neither a requirement nor a condition of treatment participation. Clients often set their individual goals, which may or may not be total abstinence or may involve a more stepped approach toward abstinence.

In the relapse prevention approach, relapse is expressly discussed, focusing on events preceding the initial use of a substance, or "lapse," as well as what happens after a lapse. According to the relapse prevention model, a lapse is often followed by what is referred to as the "abstinence violation effect," or the self-blame, guilt, and loss of control that is typically experienced after the violation of a self-imposed rule (e.g., an individual may have thought "I have already failed, so I may as well go all the way"; Curry, Marlatt, & Gordon, 1987). This puts the individual at an increased risk of relapse. Relapse prevention emphasizes the danger of a lapse while encouraging individuals to recognize that they still have the choice to cope effectively following a lapse and to return to their initial goals (Marlatt & Witkiewitz, 2005).

Similarly, although MBRP strongly supports abstinence, it is up to participants to decide what, if any, changes they choose for themselves. Because MBRP is designed as an aftercare program, participants typically have already undergone treatment, and thus may have clarified their own goals or have had to comply with the goals of the legal system or the treatment program. The MBRP approach does not necessarily address "goals," however. The mindfulness-based practices encourage individuals to become familiar with their thoughts, emotional reactions, and behavioral patterns. For some this might result in a reduction in or alteration of their pattern of use, and for others it may result in complete abstinence. A lapse is seen as a common occurrence in the change process and represents a learning opportunity rather than a failure or a return to square one. The overarching focus of MBRP on increasing awareness, however, allows flexibility to consider the individual needs and objectives of varied treatment programs.

Navigation of these differences can be challenging, and may be especially evident in Session 6's discussion of the relapse cycle, where a lapse, or single use, is differentiated from a return to the relapse cycle. It is often useful at this point to turn the discussion over to the group rather than presenting a certain model or theory of relapse. Participants can share experiences of previous relapses and the specific events leading up to an initial lapse. This often initiates a more organic discussion of various points in the chain of events where there might have been opportunities to "pause," stepping out of the "automatic" mode and breaking the chain of habitual behavior. The approach is collaborative and tends to lead to a more natural and relevant discussion of the powerful role of thoughts in the relapse process, specifically following an initial lapse, and the potential benefits of mindfulness in changing this pattern.

Fundamentally, both the 12-step and MBRP approaches begin with a realization that one's present behavioral and cognitive habits are causing suffering, and that the "refuge" of substance use is ultimately a false one. Both programs encourage developing wisdom to discern what we can and cannot control and an acceptance of that which is not in our control. Finally, the programs similarly encourage recognition of factors that increase vulnerability to relapse or other problematic habitual behaviors, such as states of body and mind (e.g., lonely, tired). They appreciate the mind's tendency to attach to unhelpful patterns (e.g., "resentments" in the 12-step approach or judgments and stories in MBRP) that ultimately cause more suffering and increase risk of relapse.

LOGISTICS

In addition to the theoretical and stylistic challenges that may arise, there are also some practical challenges of conducting MBRP, especially in the context of a treatment agency. These include scheduling, legalities of reporting use, participant motivation, and barriers to practice. We offer here some issues that we have encountered and about which we are often asked.

Time

For those working within an agency, there may be limitations to the length and timing of the groups. Two hours is usually sufficient to cover the material outlined for each session; however, a shorter duration limits either the practices or the discussions, whereas an additional 15 to 30 minutes allows for a more in-depth exploration of the experiences and observations that arise in group. When scheduling permits, we recommend experimenting with longer sessions when possible (2.5-hour sessions are often used in MBSR and MBCT). Another common experience is difficulty scheduling a half or full day of mindfulness during the course, as recommended by both MBSR and MBCT. As any mindfulness practitioner who has been on intensive retreat knows, there are many merits to sustained periods of mindfulness. However, constraints of scheduling and space for those working in agencies or other institutional settings may not allow for this opportunity.

Legal Issues

Participants who are court mandated to complete substance abuse treatment often have complex motivations and can present challenges to open discussion of substance use occurring during the course. This can detract from the honesty, openness, and nonjudgmental stance that MBRP is designed to cultivate and model. Additionally, it may prevent some participants from returning to the group following an instance of use. Ideally, groups include discussion of lapses that occur during the course of the treatment, allowing participants an experience of acceptance and support, even in the event of a lapse in abstinence. This provides an opportunity to observe the tendency of the mind in such a situation and to reinforce, as much as possible, letting go of judgment and beginning again.

Home Practice

Full participation in group sessions and in home practice is essential to the integration of MBRP practices into daily life. Facilitation and support of daily meditation and regular group attendance are thus core emphases throughout the 8 weeks. Participants often rely heavily on the audio-recorded guided meditations for the first several weeks, after which many continue practice in silence without the guided instructions. Although previously recorded meditation CDs, such as those created by Jon Kabat-Zinn (2002), are an option, creating unique recordings has many potential advantages. For instance, participants often prefer to hear the familiar voices of their facilitators, and consistency between the in-session and recorded meditation instructions may support overall engagement with the practice. Additionally, participants often express preference for a female voice to guide them through the meditation instructions. Finally, it can be useful to offer meditations of different lengths of time, and recording one's own CDs allows for inclusion of recorded instructions for lovingkindness, or "metta," meditation and practices tailored more specifically to cravings and urges. Thus, we encourage facilitators to record their own CDs whenever possible. As an example, we have typically offered four CDs that include the following:

- CD 1: Body Scan
- CD 2: Breath Meditation, Mountain Meditation, SOBER Breathing Space, Urge Surfing
- CD 3: Sitting Meditation (with awareness of breath, sound, sensation, thought, emotion), Movement, Silence with Bells (bells at 10, 20, and 30 minutes for those wishing to practice in silence)
- CD 4: Lovingkindness Meditation

Participants' living situations may present additional barriers to daily practice. For example, they may be housed in challenging or unstable living situations, with consequent difficulties in finding time and space for meditation practice. We have loaned inexpensive playback equipment in such cases and have spent time in groups generating ideas for practice times and places. Although living conditions may remain a real barrier for some participants, many are able to work within the bounds of their situations and find creative ways to integrate formal practice into their daily lives, for example, practicing while on long bus rides or retreating to libraries or even their parked car, where they can take a break from the chaos of their homes to practice. Some agencies and clinics have designated on-site daily practice time and space to support participants' practice.

Attendance

Regular attendance in groups is essential to learning the mindfulness-based skills and practices. Not surprisingly, participants unable to attend sessions are often less engaged in subsequent sessions. We have found this especially true of attendance in the first session; those who miss the initial session never quite "catch up" or engage as fully in the group as other members. Despite attempts to "fill them in" on the material and practices covered in previous missed sessions, we found that there were layers to the practice and experience that could only be integrated in "real time," and that the shared experiences and discussions of the group were valuable and essential for a richer understanding of and engagement with the practices.

Gender and Group Size

The MBRP structured protocol does not specifically address group composition by gender; however, it is an issue worthy of consideration when organizing a group.

Having facilitated both mixed-gender and gender-segregated groups, our experience indicates that some participants, particularly females with a history of interpersonal trauma, may benefit more from gender-specific groups.

The ideal group size in our experience is 6 to 12 participants, although we have facilitated groups of as many as 18. A larger group size may result in decreased time for each individual to share her or his experiences, questions, and concerns, and may present a challenge for facilitators to complete all of the intended exercises while providing adequate time for inquiry, which is an essential aspect of the program. On the other hand, a small group (fewer than six) means fewer opportunities for participants to learn from others' experiences, which provides a tremendous amount of support and validation.

Precourse Meetings

In our efforts to increase retention and therapeutic alliance, coupled with the MBSR and MBCT practice of conducting initial interviews with prospective group members, we have found that holding brief individual meetings with each participant before the course can be helpful in assessing and clarifying expectations, providing a rationale for the significant commitment the course requires, and allowing an opportunity for prospective participants to raise questions or concerns. We typically review the basic structure of the course (e.g., schedule, expectations, attendance), highlight the importance of home practice, and inquire about motivation and anticipated barriers to participation. It is helpful to elicit from individuals their own motivations and commitment rather than attempt to "sell" them on the course. Even these brief meetings seem to enhance interest and commitment, increase rapport, and improve attendance.

ISSUES TO CONSIDER

Although we have learned substantial and invaluable lessons throughout the process of designing, training, implementing, and evaluating MBRP, there are several areas and issues that we continue to explore, several of which are discussed next.

Lovingkindness

Metta, or lovingkindness, is a core practice in the Theravada tradition, where vipassana meditation has its roots. The practice typically involves bringing one's attention to a set of phrases intended to cultivate an attitude of friendliness and kindness toward oneself, friends and loved ones, strangers or "neutral" people, those who are challenging, and finally toward all beings. Although both MBSR and MBCT include several other fundamental techniques and practices central to vipassana meditation, explicit practices of metta are typically not included. Similarly, we did not include metta practice in the initial development of MBRP. It wasn't until we had conducted several groups that we began to question this exclusion. Self-judgment and self-criticism are pervasive and palpable among individuals with substance abuse histories. Not only do these individuals often internalize the judgment and stigma they have experienced from society and family, but they frequently have great difficulty forgiving themselves for negative consequences that have arisen as a result of their substance use. Thus, we began to appreciate the need for cultivation of friendliness and warmth toward oneself as central to recovery and healing. We began to include aspects of metta and forgiveness in several of the meditation instructions and a formal metta practice in the final two sessions. Although there is not yet empirical support for this element of the program, we strongly recommend its inclusion.

Physical Posture

Posture during practices, while seemingly minor, can be an important issue to consider. Although some participants may choose to sit in chairs because of physical concerns, many may choose to use cushions, mats, or pillows on the floor. Sitting on the floor often creates an atmosphere of familiarity and shared experience, shifting the role of the facilitators from authorities to fellow meditation practitioners. However, it may also inadvertently foster the notion that mindfulness practice requires adopting a special posture and is something that is practiced "on the cushion" rather than in daily life. Sitting or lying down on the floor may also increase drowsiness or laxity in posture. Having a single zafu or similar cushion placed underneath each chair may allow experimentation with sitting postures while also maintaining some of the formality of practice. We recommend that facilitators experiment in their groups and find what feels best suited to themselves and their participants.

Working with Trauma

The usefulness and safety of working with individuals with a history of trauma is a common and important issue. Creating a safe environment is imperative for all participants, but it is especially crucial for those with trauma histories or for whom safety and trust are significant concerns. Above all, the intention of the practice needs to be kept at the forefront: to cultivate clear seeing and compassion. We are observing our experiences—particularly those that are painful—with curiosity, presence, and gentleness, so as to practice a different way of relating to them. Although often uncomfortable and challenging, these practices should never feel threatening and are thus best fostered in a safe, supported context. Individualizing practices to support this is fine. Sitting in chairs or keeping eyes open during sitting and body scan practices should always be offered as options. For participants with a history of trauma, lying down, especially in the first session, can be overwhelming and can undermine the sense of safety and comfort necessary for these groups. Some participants may practice all meditations with eyes open or may prefer walking meditation over sitting practices. Participants can choose the form of practice that is best suited to their needs.

"Closed" versus "Rolling" Groups

As currently designed, MBRP is delivered in a "closed" group format, with all participants beginning together at Session 1 and finishing together at Session 8. The practices are designed to build upon one another, and thus sessions are kept in sequence. However, we and some of our colleagues have been experimenting with different formats—for example, admitting new participants at Week 4, with the addition of an introductory session exclusively for the new participants (Brewer et al., 2009), or implementing a "rolling" course design, wherein participants can enter or exit the group at any point. Although a closed group format, with members experiencing the full 8-week course together, offers many benefits, a rolling format may permit more clients to participate in the course and allow "experienced" participants to inform and support the newer participants. We look forward to learning from our own and our colleagues' future experiences with these various formats.

RESEARCH ON MBRP

Our research team at the University of Washington's Addictive Behaviors Research Center recently conducted a randomized controlled pilot trial comparing the 8-week MBRP course outlined in this guide with the standard aftercare groups at a local community treatment agency (see Bowen et al., 2009, for a full report). The agency's standard aftercare groups were aligned with a 12-step philosophy and included both process-oriented and psychoeducational groups. Discussions included topics such as grief and loss, assertiveness, self-esteem, goal setting, rational thinking, and relapse prevention skills. All study participants ($N = 168$) had recently completed intensive inpatient or outpatient treatment at the agency for a variety of alcohol and other drug use disorders, and they represented a diverse cross-section of the urban treatment-involved population. Several of the agency clients were homeless, and many were legally mandated to receive treatment. The study sample was predominantly male (64%), with a mean age of 40 years.

The majority of the sample self-identified as Caucasian (52%), African American (30%), or Native American (10%). Approximately 72% had at least a high school diploma. However, 41% were unemployed, and 62% earned less than $4,999 per year. Although many of these individuals were polysubstance users, the primary drug of choice was alcohol (45%), followed closely by cocaine/crack (36%) and methamphetamines (14%).

Study participants were randomly assigned to either take part in an 8-week MBRP course or to remain in their current standard aftercare groups for the duration of the 8-week program. All participants, regardless of assignment, were encouraged to continue to attend additional self-help groups as recommended by the treatment agency. Following completion of the 8-week program, MBRP participants returned to their standard aftercare groups. Those assigned to standard aftercare were given the opportunity to attend the MBRP course free of charge upon completion of the study.

At multiple time points throughout the study, participants were asked to complete several assessments. They gave retrospective reports of their substance use in the 60 days prior to admission into treatment, at the end of treatment (immediately following the 8-week program), and finally at 2 and 4 months immediately following treatment. Assessments of consequences related to use, craving, depression, anxiety, and levels of mindfulness and acceptance were also included at these time points.

An important goal of this first randomized controlled trial of MBRP was to evaluate the program's feasibility: Would it be well tolerated by participants? Would they attend the treatment sessions and engage in daily meditation practice and the assigned exercises to be completed outside of sessions? Our results indicated that MBRP participants reported attending an average of 65% of treatment sessions. The majority (86%) reported engaging in meditation practices immediately following the treatment program, and a substantial portion (54%) continued meditation practice for at least 4 months after treatment completion (for an average of 4.74 days per week and almost 30 minutes per day). The results of a feedback questionnaire administered during the final session were positive. Participants rated the course as highly important to them (average rating of 8.3 on a scale of 0–10) and reported a high likelihood of continuing both formal meditation practices, including the body scan, sitting, and yoga (8.9 out of 10), and informal meditation practices, such as urge surfing and "breathing spaces" (8.9 out of 10).

In addition to the apparent acceptability and feasibility of the program, the outcome data suggested promising results. MBRP participants demonstrated significantly greater decreases in craving over the 4-month follow-up period compared with those in standard aftercare. They also reported greater increases in acceptance and in the tendency to act with awareness. These changes are consistent with several of the core goals of MBRP, including acceptance of both pleasant and unpleasant experience and heightened awareness of triggers, with the goal of stepping out of well-practiced patterns of reactive behavior into more skillful behavioral choices.

Finally, participants in both conditions demonstrated an overall reduction in days of alcohol and drug use. However, days of substance use were decreased to a significantly greater extent among the MBRP group, with an average of 0.06 days of use over the 8-week course compared with 2.57 days of use for standard after-care participants. These differences continued to be significant 2 months following treatment (2.08 days of use for MBRP participants vs. 5.43 days of use for standard aftercare participants), but appeared to diminish at 4 months, with days of use for the MBRP group returning to similar levels as for the standard aftercare group.

Although encouraged by these results, we have given significant consideration to addressing the attenuation of treatment effects at the final follow-up time point. This may be attributable to the design of the study, which required MBRP participants to return to standard aftercare groups on completion of the 8-week MBRP program. These standard groups did not typically include continuation of the mindfulness practices and perspectives learned in MBRP. Further, the standard groups may have involved practices that were counter to those in the MBRP group, and thus may have been confusing or contradictory for participants. For instance, rather than encouraging acceptance and awareness of cravings and urges, these groups may have emphasized strategies such as distraction and avoidance of unpleasant experience. This led our research team to consider offering continued support and maintenance of the approaches learned in MBRP. As most meditation practitioners discover, it is extraordinarily challenging to maintain a practice independently, in the absence of a teacher or group of fellow practitioners. Without a community and opportunities for supported practice, it is easy to fall back into the habitual patterns of mind and into previous reactive or "automatic" behaviors. Thus, it is our recommendation that future applications and modifications of MBRP consider the addition of ongoing weekly or monthly sitting groups or other continued support as part of the treatment program.

Overall results of this study offer empirical promise for MBRP as an aftercare treatment and support the theoretical framework behind the use of mindfulness meditation for substance use disorders. Participant attendance, continued meditation practice, and positive course ratings support the feasibility, tolerability, and appeal of the program. The increases in awareness and acceptance and decreases in craving and substance use provide initial evidence for its efficacy. Results from this study complement those from related studies. A pilot study conducted by Zgierska et al. (2008) evaluated the feasibility and efficacy of MBRP for 19 alcohol-dependent individuals following intensive inpatient treatment. Similar to the results of our study, participants reported a high degree of satisfaction with the program and compliance with the daily meditation practices both during and 2 months after course completion. Additionally, participants reported reductions in alcohol consumption, increases in mindfulness, and decreases in several potential triggers for relapse, including depression, anxiety, stress, and craving. This study also assessed several biological markers of stress and health and found modest reductions indicative of greater health and well-being.

Brewer and colleagues (2009) recently compared the effects of mindfulness training and CBT among individuals with alcohol and/or cocaine use disorders. Following random assignment to and completion of treatment, both the mindfulness training and CBT groups participated in a personalized stress provocation task followed by self-report measures as well psychophysiological measures of skin conductance, heart rate, and heart rate variability. Results suggested that the mindfulness group showed reduced psychological and physiological responses to stress compared with the CBT group.

Taken together, these studies offer compelling preliminary evidence for MBRP. Further research replicating these findings, evaluating benefits of ongoing post-treatment support, identifying mechanisms of change, and assessing for whom this treatment is most beneficial, will offer further support for and a more nuanced assessment of the program. The chapters that follow describe the protocol as implemented in the discussed trial. We expect that MBRP will continue to evolve as future studies clarify strengths or shortcomings and as application to specific populations and settings call for adaptations. We look forward to its evolution.

PART II

Facilitator's Guide

As DESCRIBED IN PART I OF THIS BOOK, this program is designed to be facilitated by therapists with an established foundation in mindfulness meditation, an ongoing daily practice, and, ideally, formal training in MBRP, MBSR, or MBCT. We suggest that readers begin with Part I before continuing on to the treatment guide.

The following chapters offer a framework for those wishing to facilitate MBRP groups. Although we have included scripts for the meditation practices, these are intended as suggestions or examples to help facilitators become comfortable with guiding meditations. As mentioned in the Introduction, a facilitator's engagement and presence in leading each of these practices is an opportunity to model the embodiment of the qualities of spontaneity, presence, and openness to one's own arising experiences. This offers authenticity that can be lost when following a script and exemplifies the "trust in experience" and present-centeredness that are foundational to MBRP. We thus encourage facilitators to participate in all meditation exercises while leading them, guiding from their own experience rather than simply giving instructions or reading from a script.

OVERVIEW OF SESSIONS

The following chapters outline each of the eight sessions (see Table II.1). Chapters include an overview of the topics and themes included in each session, a detailed discussion of the practices and exercises, and of the experiences and challenges that often arise. We include excerpted dialogue to clarify and aid in the illustration

TABLE II.1 Sessions in the MBRP Program

◆ Session 1: Automatic Pilot and Relapse

◆ Session 2: Awareness of Triggers and Craving

◆ Session 3: Mindfulness in Daily Life

◆ Session 4: Mindfulness in High-Risk Situations

◆ Session 5: Acceptance and Skillful Action

◆ Session 6: Seeing Thoughts as Thoughts

◆ Session 7: Self-Care and Lifestyle Balance

◆ Session 8: Social Support and Continuing Practice

of themes, practices, and discussions. The specific exercises and handouts listed and discussed in each session are included at the end of each chapter.

Although each session has a central theme, the sessions are intended to build upon the previous weeks' materials and practices. Similar to MBSR and MBCT, the course begins with an experiential introduction to the tendency toward "automatic pilot." Exercises and discussions in the first three sessions center on this theme. By bringing awareness to this deeply habitual tendency, and through specific practices designed to bring attention to the present, participants begin stepping out of this automatic mode, both in session and in their daily lives. Awareness of the role of automatic pilot in relapse is also discussed in these initial sessions. Sessions 4 to 6 explore the application of practices learned thus far to situations in which participants might be at increased risk of relapse or reactive behavior. These sessions identify individual risk profiles and involve integrating mindfulness skills into these situations. Finally, Sessions 7 and 8 widen the lens, looking at the bigger picture of creating and maintaining a lifestyle that will support both recovery and mindfulness practice.

The first formal practice introduced in the course is the body scan exercise. Throughout the 8 weeks, this focus on the body remains central and is revisited through practices such as walking meditation, mindful movement, and inquiry. The body is the first foundation of mindfulness, providing a dependable way of bringing attention into the present moment. This practice also presents an opportunity to observe how the mind responds to uncomfortable experiences, learning how to "be with" discomfort and craving rather than reacting in habitual and often destructive ways. The practices gradually progress to working with emotional discomfort, encouraging greater gentleness and acceptance of one's internal experience. Once participants have had some experience observing sensations and emotional states, they are introduced to the observation of thoughts as objects of awareness. In the final sessions, practices centered on the active cultivation of kindness and self-compassion are introduced.

BEGINNING AND ENDING EACH SESSION

In addition to planning the specific structure and preparing materials for each session, a period of meditation before the start of each session can promote greater awareness and presence in the group and a fuller embodiment of the qualities we are encouraging in our participants. Entering the room in a calmer, clearer state of mind fosters a space that is grounding, safe, and accepting.

Sessions can easily end with a flurry of papers, scheduling details, and rushed gathering of belongings. Continuation of practice into daily life can be further supported by inviting participants at the close of each session to stop wherever they are, without the need to shift into any special posture, and take a brief pause to focus on the breath, on sounds, or on what is happening in their bodies. They can then be encouraged to stay with this awareness as they gather their things and move into the rest of their day or evening.

Automatic Pilot and Relapse

Life is not lost by dying
Life is lost minute by minute
Day by dragging day
In all the small and uncaring ways
—STEPHEN VINCENT BENET

MATERIALS

- ◆ Raisins (or dried cranberries), bowl, spoon
- ◆ Body scan CDs
- ◆ Binders with handouts
- ◆ Bell
- ◆ Whiteboard/markers
- ◆ Handout 1.1: Overview of Sessions
- ◆ Handout 1.2: Definition of Mindfulness
- ◆ Handout 1.3: Session 1 Theme and Home Practice: Automatic Pilot and Relapse
- ◆ Handout 1.4: Daily Practice Tracking Sheet

THEME

When we experience cravings and urges to use alcohol or drugs, we often engage in reactive behaviors, acting on them without full awareness of what is occurring and what the consequences will be. This first session introduces the idea of "automatic pilot," or acting without awareness, and discusses the relationship between automatic pilot and relapse. We begin by using mindful awareness to recognize this tendency, and then learn ways to begin shifting from habitual and often self-defeating behavior to observation of what is happening in our minds and bodies without "automatically" reacting. This session uses the raisin exercise to introduce mindful awareness and contrast it to automatic pilot. Body scan practice is then introduced as a way of bringing attention to present-moment experiences of the body.

GOALS

◆ Introduce "automatic pilot" and bring awareness to how unaware we often are.

◆ Introduce foundations and practices of MBRP.

◆ Introduce mindfulness as a means of becoming aware of the patterns of the mind.

◆ Introduce the body scan as a way of bringing awareness to physical expression.

SESSION OUTLINE

◆ Introductions

◆ Expectations for Group and Rules for Confidentiality and Privacy

◆ Group Structure and Format

◆ Raisin Exercise (Practice 1.1)/Automatic Pilot and Relapse

◆ What Is Mindfulness?

◆ Body Scan Meditation (Practice 1.2)

◆ Home Practice

◆ Closing

HOME PRACTICE

◆ Body scan 6 out of 7 days

◆ Mindfulness of a daily activity

◆ Daily Practice Tracking Sheet

The primary intention of this first session is to introduce some basics of mindfulness practice, to offer an experiential sense of the automatic pilot mode, and to begin discriminating between automatic versus mindful awareness. The session also introduces the relationship between automatic or reactive behavior and relapse. Participants experience the basic components of mindful awareness through exercises that encourage slowing down, paying attention to present-moment experience, and observing the mind and the different senses.

INTRODUCTIONS

In this first session, facilitators set the tone for the group and create a space that supports exploration and presence. To emphasize the experiential nature of the course, it is helpful to keep the beginning logistics and explanations brief. Introductions, too, are typically kept to name and (briefly) reason for participation in the course. During this first round of introductions, participants often describe outward motivations, such as the need to meet requirements of probation or in the context of a research study, the payment they may receive for participation. Although these may be very real motivators for some, a second round of inquiry can be useful in tapping a deeper value or intention that may be more sustaining. Thus, facilitators may initiate a second round of introductions by asking participants to take a moment to reflect on what is really important to them in their lives (e.g., connection with family, living a full, rich life). This may be facilitated by asking the following questions: What do you most value about being here? If treatment could really help you have the life you wanted, what would shift?" Again, comments should be kept brief.

EXPECTATIONS FOR GROUP AND RULES
FOR CONFIDENTIALITY AND PRIVACY

In the discussion of confidentiality and basic group guidelines, we often ask participants what factors are necessary to ensure a sense of safety and comfort and what will facilitate their participation and engagement in the course. Key components that often arise are consistency in attendance, notifying facilitators in advance of an absence, confidentiality, commitment to the work and the process, honesty, a nonjudgmental attitude, and other issues involving basic respect for other group members' needs and experience. Having this conversation up front strengthens group cohesion and fosters an attitude of respect, commitment, and engagement in making the group most conducive to full participation.

GROUP STRUCTURE AND FORMAT

Basic structure and logistics of the course, such as times, breaks, and so on, are important to describe, and also best kept as brief as possible so that the experiential nature of the program is emphasized in this beginning session. It is helpful to let participants know that discussions will focus on present experiences rather than on stories, ideas, conceptual thinking, or "processing." Throughout the course, facilitators might redirect the discussion, reminding group members to return to present experience or using the bell to suggest taking a pause and gathering attention if the group has strayed from the intended focus. Facilitators explain that sessions are rich in material and exercises, and that each person may not have the opportunity to share his or her experience following every exercise. Given that similar themes and exercises are covered repeatedly (Handout 1.1), all participants will have a chance at some point to share their experiences.

It is suggested that, as best they can, participants suspend judgments or ideas about the value of these practices until the end of the course, bringing a willingness to experience whatever arises with curiosity and openness. At the end of the 8 weeks, they will have the opportunity to assess the value of the practice in their lives and can choose whether or not to continue. As long as they are committed to attending the course, they are asked to "jump in" and to participate fully.

In beginning discussions of home practice, it is useful for participants to understand that the in-session practices are only an introduction and that, although they will inevitably learn from these alone, this course is most powerful when these practices are integrated into their daily lives, which takes some commitment and effort, especially in the beginning. Practicing the daily meditations and completing the worksheets outside of group is essential, as is attendance at all eight sessions. Each session builds on themes and exercises from previous weeks; thus, attending group each week and doing one's best to engage in the home practices are crucial to the program.

RAISIN EXERCISE/AUTOMATIC PILOT AND RELAPSE

Each session begins with a mindfulness exercise, followed by a discussion in which experiences and themes are elicited from participants. As presented in the Introductions section, discussions are guided using open-ended questions and facilitated with a nonjudgmental, present-centered stance that is reflective of the practice itself.

Similar to the MBSR and MBCT programs, the first experiential exercise in MBRP involves mindfully observing and eating a single raisin (Practice 1.1).* The raisin exercise is a wonderful illustration of mindfully engaging in an activity that we have likely performed hundreds of times, often without much awareness. Further, eating is a visceral experience that allows awareness of sensations in the body as well as reactions of either "liking/desire" or "disliking/aversion." The act of slowing down and paying close attention to the various sensations, thoughts, urges, and even emotions involved in this simple activity illustrates how a typically automatic behavior, when observed, offers a rich array of experiences. It allows participants to experience the difference between mindful attention and a more automatic mode and provides an opportunity to discuss the relationship among automatic pilot, addiction, and relapse.

Following the exercise, facilitators inquire about individuals' experiences, including sensations, thoughts, feelings, urges, as well as any reactions to those experiences, such as judgment, aversion, or pleasure. The primary focus is on the direct experience, with facilitators continually redirecting where necessary. Participants reliably comment on how they have never "really tasted" a raisin or observed the nuances of it or how they typically eat a handful without even being aware that they have consumed them. This often progresses to discussion of the parallels between this experience and blindly following a craving or an urge without attention to the numerous steps and reactions involved in the downward spiral.

This is illustrated in the following example:

FACILITATOR: What did people notice in doing this exercise?

PARTICIPANT 1: I noticed I started thinking about how this raisin was alive at one time, and noticing it had seeds in it. My mind automatically went to "grape—this was a grape. Now it's a raisin."

FACILITATOR: So thoughts arose about the history of this object. It seems like you noticed some of the more subtle properties of the object as well, like the seeds.

PARTICIPANT 2: I noticed the color, a beautiful red. It looked like one side was shriveled with tiny, tiny seeds and the other side was shiny. Then my mind went off to pretending I was beaming information back to another planet. Then my mind came back. I was excited when you said, "Put it in your mouth."

FACILITATOR: So you noticed a lot of different things. The color and texture

---

*In some of our groups, we have substituted a dried cranberry because raisins may have associations with wine for some of our participants. Although this association may offer a rich opportunity for paying attention to the experience of craving, we intend to keep this first introduction simple. Mindful observation of craving is addressed later in the program.

of the object, the tendency of the mind to wander off into a fantasy or thought. Also seems like you were aware of that, and were able to bring your attention back to the moment. And then you noticed a feeling of anticipation or desire.

PARTICIPANT 2: Once I bit into it, though, I didn't like the way it tasted.

FACILITATOR: When you say you didn't like how it tasted, what happened? How did you experience "not liking"?

PARTICIPANT 2: When it got to the back of my throat before I swallowed, there was a reaction in my mouth, my throat and mouth, that was not a pleasant taste, and I thought "I don't like it."

FACILITATOR: So both a physical reaction and the thought "I don't like this."

PARTICIPANT 3: I had the thought that I wanted some more.

FACILITATOR: Ahh. So an awareness that this experience would end, and a desire for it to continue, to have more. And were there any sensations that you noticed along with that, the thought of wanting more?

PARTICIPANT 3: Yeah, I noticed my mouth watering.

In this discussion, the facilitator highlights the direct sensory experience, gently redirecting comments that wander into stories or reactions. The facilitator also distinguishes between thoughts and sensations. The intention is for participants not only to bring their awareness to present-moment experience but also to become aware of the tendency of the mind to wander away from the moment and to learn to gently guide it back without judgment. Further, the idea of thoughts being mere "objects of awareness" rather than facts or truths is introduced.

FACILITATOR: So let me ask: All these details, is this something you would typically notice when eating a raisin?

PARTICIPANT 1: No, I never have before. I'd just eat it.

FACILITATOR: How is this different than how you normally eat a raisin?

PARTICIPANT 1: I just shove a bunch in my mouth.

FACILITATOR: So speed is part of it; you usually eat faster.

PARTICIPANT 1: Yeah, especially when I come home at night I just eat, and I'm not usually paying attention.

FACILITATOR: So your mind is maybe elsewhere, not on what you are actually doing. Maybe reviewing the day or thinking about what's for dessert or worrying about tomorrow's appointment. The eating is automatic.

PARTICIPANT 1: I already know what I'm eating so I don't pay attention, I don't look at it. I've done this a thousand times.

PARTICIPANT 2: Yeah, I've never slowed down like that, looked at it, felt it, appreciated it.

PARTICIPANT 1: It's kind of like when you've been locked up [incarcerated] and you finally get your freedom back. When you have it, you don't appreciate it. But when it's taken away, you understand freedom again, you suddenly appreciate everything, you notice everything you used to just take for granted.

FACILITATOR: All these things you used to take for granted you suddenly notice and appreciate—even these so-called "little" things. There may be some connection between that and freedom for you—interesting.

So you mentioned this idea of it being automatic, you've done it a thousand times before, not paying attention. Every week's session has a theme, and this week's theme is exactly what we're discussing here: "automatic pilot." Can you think of other examples of times in your life when you're on automatic pilot?

PARTICIPANT 3: Driving to work—it's like, "What happened back there?" That whole time disappeared.

The prior dialogue again illustrates the facilitator's intention to elicit ideas and themes from participants when possible rather than "teaching" the core themes or attempting to stress the importance of the practices. By asking how the experience with the raisin contrasts with their typical way of doing things, facilitators encourage participants to become more aware of their tendency to live on automatic pilot. In our experience, these key themes reliably arise from discussion, with some gentle direction, open questions, and a focus on present-moment experience. This gradually moves to the distinction between this and typical experience and, finally, the relationship of this experience to relapse. We have also found it helpful to draw all participants into the group, often highlighting the "nonpersonal" nature of an individual's experience by asking whether others in the group experienced something similar or different. Typically, experiences are shared by several group members. Finally, the facilitator brings the exercise into the context of relapse:

FACILITATOR: So why are we doing this exercise in a relapse-prevention group? How do you think this might be related to relapse or addiction?

PARTICIPANT1: When you start drinking, you're already on automatic pilot. It's something you've done a million times. You already know where you're going to go, what you're going to do. It's not conscious.

PARTICIPANT 2: For me it happens way before I use the actual substance. It might be a month previous, a little thought pops into my mind or I do something . . . like I used to sell drugs but not use them. But in the scheme of things I knew I was going to use eventually. It was a huge lie to myself. If you don't stop and pay attention, you can be on that road without seeing it.

FACILITATOR: So slowing down and noticing where we are and what our minds are doing. Bringing some awareness to what is happening in the moment might help us make more skillful choices.

Throughout this course, we will practice awareness of sensations, thoughts, and emotions, specifically in relation to cravings and relapse. We will practice new ways to relate to these experiences, especially difficult ones, so that we don't just default to our habitual ways. We are not trying to get rid of all difficult experiences; we are learning to relate to them differently so we have more choice in how we respond. So that maybe they don't have as much control over us.

WHAT IS MINDFULNESS?

The raisin exercise allows participants the opportunity to explore mindful attention and, based on their own experience, begin a discussion of mindfulness. Following the exercise, we ask participants to describe, from what they have experienced thus far, what "mindfulness" means. Participants often point to qualities of awareness, choice, present-centered focus or "being in the moment," ability to stop habitual responses, and feelings of connection. It can be helpful to write these on the whiteboard and note themes that emerge. We usually follow this with a handout (1.2) of Kabat-Zinn's description of mindfulness: "Mindfulness means paying attention in a particular way: on purpose, in the present moment and non-judgmentally."

The aspects of paying attention and focusing on present-moment experience have often been offered by participants in the discussion. The quality of gentleness and kindness toward one's experience, however, frequently goes unmentioned. We have found it useful to highlight this aspect of the practice repeatedly throughout the course: Mindfulness is not only about paying attention to what is occurring but also about having compassion and, as best we can, adopting a nonjudgmental stance toward whatever is arising. Participants inevitably experience judgment toward themselves and their experiences, including their ability to engage in the practice. We are practicing noticing with curiosity rather than evaluation or judgment, both by modeling this stance toward whatever participants raise in session and by explicitly reminding them to be gentle with themselves. It is helpful to return to this conversation throughout the course, continually encouraging participants to bring a spacious, curious awareness to all experience regardless of whether it is pleasant or unpleasant. For example, when aversive reactions to the raisin exercise arise, it can be an excellent first opportunity to highlight awareness of aversion and to model a curious and nonjudgmental stance even toward that which we don't like.

BODY SCAN MEDITATION

Similar to the MBSR and MBCT programs, the first formal meditation practice in the course is the body scan meditation (Practice 1.2). In the vipassana, or "insight," meditative tradition from which this practice originates, awareness of the body is described as the first foundation of mindfulness. The practice then expands to include awareness of other levels of experience, including emotions and mental events. Once again, we have found it imperative in this exercise to emphasize openness to and curiosity about any and all experiences that arise while practicing the body scan, disabusing expectations about what one should or shouldn't experience and reminding participants that it is simply about learning to pay attention to experience, whatever it may be.

In the context of relapse prevention, the practice of paying attention to physical experience can be especially valuable, because experiences of reactivity, cravings, and urges often manifest physically before the subsequent chain of thoughts or reactions. When in automatic pilot mode, we often lose contact with the immediate physical experience. Thus, coming back to physical sensations is a way of reconnecting with present experience and can be a first step in shifting from habitual, reactive behavior to making more mindful choices.

Because this is the first "formal" practice in which participants engage, it is helpful to offer the choice to either lie down on the floor or sit in chairs, with eyes either open or closed, depending on participants' level of safety and comfort. It is also important to spend a few moments encouraging participants to find a posture that is balanced and stable, particularly if sitting, that they can maintain for about 25 to 30 minutes.

In the inquiry following the body scan, participants typically express a range of responses, from experiences of peace and relaxation to restlessness and physical discomfort. The following is an example of the type of discussion that often follows this practice:

FACILITATOR: What were people's observations and experiences?

PARTICIPANT 1: That was really relaxing.

FACILITATOR: What did you notice in your body or mind that was "relaxing"?

PARTICIPANT 1: Just like a sensation of release and breathing more deeply.

FACILITATOR: So release of some tension, perhaps, and the breath deepening.

PARTICIPANT 2: I noticed that early on my mind was wandering away from the area we were focusing on, but later on it wasn't drifting as much.

FACILITATOR: Ah, yes. Did anyone else notice the mind wandering off to other things?

In this example, the facilitator begins with the first level of the inquiry process by focusing on direct experience of "relaxing." The facilitator then addresses the nonpersonal nature to normalize or validate an experience that could easily elicit self-judgment or an expectation of a fully concentrated mind that does not wander. The facilitator begins with a recognition of this tendency of the mind ("Ah, yes") followed by the invitation for others to share similar experiences ("Did anyone else notice the mind wandering?"). A facilitator may even offer his or her own experience with the practice to reduce any misconceptions and to illustrate the universality of this tendency. Finally, as the discussion continues, the facilitator inquires about "mental proliferation," asking for reactions or judgments to the experience of a wandering mind. As illustrated, all levels of inquiry are not necessarily touched upon in every interaction and are not necessarily in a set order:

FACILITATOR: For those of you who noticed the mind wandering, what happened when you noticed that? What was the reaction?

PARTICIPANT 1: Well, when I found myself somewhere else, I realized that I wasn't doing what I was supposed to be doing.

FACILITATOR: So you were aware of your mind wandering, and then had a thought like, "I'm not doing what I'm supposed to be doing"?

PARTICIPANT 2: Yeah, like, "I'm doing this wrong."

FACILITATOR: So the thought, "I'm doing this wrong." Anyone else notice any judgment?

PARTICIPANT 2: Yeah, I noticed that, too.

FACILITATOR: It can be helpful to notice that "I'm doing this wrong" is a thought and gently bring your attention to the body again. As we discussed earlier, mindfulness is not about *not having* any thoughts or being perfectly concentrated, but rather about being aware of *whatever* is happening. So if the mind wanders a hundred times, we simply notice that and return to the body here in the present moment a hundred times. That is what we are practicing here: becoming aware of what our minds are doing.

There are often experiences of drowsiness and sleepiness that arise:

PARTICIPANT: I was struggling to stay awake because I was so relaxed.

FACILITATOR: Ah, yes, anyone else feel sleepy? When we lie down and close our eyes, it's often a signal for our bodies and minds to fall asleep, especially if we are tired. What did it feel like?

PARTICIPANT: I found that I would sort of drift off and then have a moment of being startled and waking up again.

FACILITATOR: Were there thoughts that you noticed?

PARTICIPANT: I thought "I need to stay awake."

FACILITATOR: So maybe a little judgment, too? It may be interesting to bring curiosity to the experience of sleepiness. "Oh, what does sleepiness feel like? What is it like to drift into and come out of sleep? What thoughts are arising about the experience?" If sleepiness arises repeatedly, it is sometimes helpful to do the practice sitting up and in a more alert posture, or open the eyes a little to let some light in—these may be things to experiment with this week.

Again, the facilitator validates the experience and provides insights and strategies based on his or her own experience while remaining curious and nonjudgmental. The balance here is delicate, offering some skillful ways of working with challenges in practice while still keeping the focus on present moment experience rather than "doing it right" or "fixing" it.

HOME PRACTICE

The first session establishes the tone and the expectation for the remainder of the course by stressing the importance of home practice, while emphasizing the nonjudgmental environment of the group (Handout 1.3). The importance of practice is sometimes best illustrated with analogies such as working daily to build a muscle, which gradually develops strength, or asking for an example of a skill at which a participant is adept and inquiring how he or she acquired that skill. We emphasize that the practice is core to the program and that the amount of benefit derived from the program is directly related to participants' commitment to the practice. This is balanced, however, with a clear message that they will not be judged or evaluated on whether or not they practice. However, they are strongly encouraged to experience the practice fully for these 8 weeks, and a core piece of this is the daily practice. Similarly, the Daily Practice Tracking Sheet (Handout 1.4) is presented as a way for participants to attend to what they are learning from the course and to note experiences that arise in the process rather than as an evaluative measure.

These tracking sheets also provide a means for facilitators to respond to concerns or barriers that arise during the week.

MINDFULNESS OF DAILY ACTIVITY

Again, in the tradition of MBSR and MBCT, one component of the home practice for this first week is for participants to bring the same qualities of attention, awareness, and curiosity, as were brought to eating the raisin, to a routine activity, such as brushing one's teeth or washing dishes. As with the raisin, the instruction is to pay attention to the activity as though experiencing it for the first time. We have typically provided participants with a few examples and then asked them to generate their own, either picking the same activity to repeat each day or choosing different activities throughout the week. This is simply a way for participants to begin integrating mindfulness into their lives, incorporating moments of awareness throughout their days. The intention is to recognize that all of these mindfulness exercises (formal and informal) are avenues toward strengthening the overall practice, thus making it more likely that the foundations provided in the course will be available during "routine" daily activities as well as in the more challenging situations.

Occasionally, a participant will ask in these beginning sessions about "mindfully" using alcohol or drugs. We often respond by addressing the typically habitual and reactive aspects of substance use. Although it is true that we can bring close attention and awareness to any experience, including using a substance, as the practice deepens there is often an awareness of all the steps that occur before using, such as the preceding cravings, thoughts, and feelings of discomfort that often trigger substance use. We might become aware of the emotion that drives these cravings, such as fear, boredom, or loneliness, and have compassion for our own suffering rather than a reactive need to fix or escape it. Further, the practice helps us see things more clearly and broaden our perspective. This clear seeing allows us to make more skillful choices, noticing ways in which we increase our suffering and learning ways to reduce it.

CLOSING

To encourage continuity of awareness, we end each session with a few moments of silence followed by the bell. The facilitator might lead a very brief exercise, such as awareness of body or breath, or just have the group sit in silence for a few moments, depending on the needs and feel of the group.

RAISIN EXERCISE
Practice 1.1

We're going to pass some objects around. Go ahead and take two or three and just hold them in the palm of your hand.

Now, I'd like to invite you to choose one of these objects and, as best you can, bring your full attention to this one object for the next few minutes. First, you might just notice which object you picked. Was there something about this one in particular that drew your attention?

Now look at this object carefully as though you have never seen anything like it. Bringing your attention to seeing it, maybe picking it up with the other hand and observing all its qualities. You might even imagine you've just arrived from another planet, and that your task is to observe this object in as much detail as possible, as though you are going to report back to your home planet all its properties.

You might feel its texture between your fingers, noticing its color and surfaces, and its unique shape.

While you are doing this, you might be aware, too, of thoughts you are having about this object, or about the exercise, or about how you are doing in the exercise. You might notice feelings, too, like pleasure or maybe dislike for this object or this exercise. Just noticing these thoughts or feelings as well and, as best you can, bringing your attention back to simply exploring this object.

You might bring this object up under your nose and inhale, noticing if it has a smell.

You might even bring it to your ear and squish it a little and see if it has a sound. And now taking another look at it.

And now slowly bringing this object up to your lips, aware of the arm moving the hand to position it correctly. And then gently placing the object against your lips, sensing how it feels there. Holding it there for a moment, aware of the sensations and any reactions. Maybe there's anticipation or the mouth beginning to salivate.

And now placing this object on the tongue, and pausing here to feel what this object feels like in the mouth. The surfaces, texture, even the temperature of this object. Now beginning with just one bite into this object and pausing again there. Noticing what tastes are released, if the texture has changed. Maybe the object has now become two objects.

Now chewing slowly, noting the actual taste and change in texture. Maybe noticing, too, how the tongue and jaw work together to position the object between the teeth, how the tongue knows exactly where to position it as you chew.

And when you feel ready to swallow, watching that impulse to swallow. Maybe pausing before swallowing to notice the urge. Then, as you swallow the object, as best you can, feeling it as it travels down the throat and into the belly.

You might even sense the body is one small object heavier.

BODY SCAN MEDITATION
Practice 1.2

Allowing your eyes to close gently. Taking a few moments to get in touch with the movement of your breath. When you are ready, bringing your attention to the physical sensations in your body, especially to the sensations of touch or pressure, where your body makes contact with the chair or the floor. On each outbreath, allowing yourself to let go, to sink a little deeper into the floor (or your chair).

The intention of this practice is not to change anything or to feel different, relaxed, or calm; this may happen or it may not. Instead, the intention of the practice is, as best you can, to bring awareness to any sensations you feel as you focus your attention on each part of the body. If you find your mind wandering, gently just bringing it back to awareness of your body.

Now bringing your awareness to the physical sensations in your abdomen, becoming aware of the sensations there as you breathe in, and as you breathe out. Taking a few minutes to feel the changing sensations, how the inbreath feels different than the outbreath.

Having connected with the sensations in the abdomen, moving the focus of your awareness now down through the body and into the toes of the left foot. Focusing on the big toe of the left foot. Noticing all the sensations in that toe. Then allowing your focus to move to each of the toes of the left foot in turn, bringing a gentle curiosity to the quality of sensations you find, perhaps noticing the sense of contact between the toes, a sense of tingling, warmth, or no particular sensation. If there are areas you can't feel, just keeping your focus there, noticing whatever you can about that area.

When you are ready, feeling or imagining the breath entering the lungs, and then going all the way down through the body, into the left foot, and to the toes of the left foot. Then, imagining the breath coming all the way back up from the toes, through the body and out through the nose. So you are sending your breath down to the left toes, then allowing it to come all the way back up through your body, and out your nose. As best you can, continuing this for a few breaths. It may be difficult to get the hang of it—just practice as best you can, approaching it playfully.

When you are ready, letting go of awareness of the toes, and bring your awareness to the sensations on the bottom of your left foot, bringing a gentle, curious awareness to the sole of the foot, feeling all the sensation there. Now bring your attention to the top of the foot, then to the ankle. Feeling the muscles, bones and tendons in the ankle. Now moving your attention up to the calf and the shin. Feeling the clothing against the skin of that area, or any sensations in the muscles. Now up into the knee. Detect as best you can all the sensations in these areas, sending your breath to each area as you move up the leg. You might think of your awareness as a spotlight, moving slowly through the body, bringing into focus any sensations in that area. Again, if there are areas where it is difficult to detect sensations, just feel as much as you can. Now bringing your attention to the left thigh. Noticing the sensations there. Maybe you feel the pressure of your leg against the chair, or places this part of the leg touches the floor if you are lying down.

Throughout this exercise, the mind will inevitably wander away from the breath and the body from time to time. That is entirely normal; it is what minds do. When you notice it, just acknowledge it, noticing where the mind has gone off to, and then gently return your attention to the part of the body.

(cont.)

42

Now sending your attention down to the right leg, through the right foot, and into the right toes. Again, picture the breath going down to the toes, then coming back up through the body and out the nose. Continue to bring awareness, and gentle curiosity, to the physical sensations, allowing whatever sensations are in the toes to just be here as they are. Notice now what you feel in the bottom of your right foot, in the top of the foot, and the ankle. Bringing your awareness now up to your calf and noticing the sensations there. Now to the right knee.

If you feel any pain or discomfort in any of these areas, just be aware of it, and practice sending the breath there, and as best you can, letting the sensations be as they are. Now gently guiding your awareness into your right thigh, noticing the sensations in this area. Then up into your hips and waist. Feeling your weight on the chair (or the floor). Now moving your focus slowly up to your abdomen. Feeling it rising and falling with each breath. Now moving your awareness into your ribcage. Just feeling as many sensations as you can. Moving that spotlight of attention around to your back—the lower back, and the upper back, feeling the places where it touches the chair or the floor. Feeling any places of tension or discomfort. Now up into your chest and your shoulders.

When you become aware of tension, or of other intense sensations in a particular part of the body, you might try "breathing into" them—using the breath to gently bring awareness right into the sensations, and as best you can, on the outbreath, letting go.

If you notice your thoughts wandering, or if you become distracted or restless, just notice that too. It's okay. Just gently guide your attention back to the sensations in your body.

Guiding your attention now down the left arm and into the fingers of the left hand. Feeling each finger and the places where they contact the chair or your body. Now up into the wrist and forearm. Noticing all the sensations here. In the elbow, upper arm, the shoulder. Notice any tension, tightness.

Now gently moving your attention across your body to the right side, down the right arm, and into the fingers of the right hand. Feeling each of them separately. Notice any tingling or urges to move them. Notice if there are fingers you are unable to feel as well as others. Now guiding your attention into the palm of the hand, and the wrist, the forearm and elbow. Now focusing on the upper arm and shoulder.

Let your attention now come into your neck. Feel where there is tightness or tension. Be aware of areas in which it is harder to detect sensation. Now bringing your focus up the back of your head. See if you can feel the hair on your head. Bringing awareness to the left ear, then over to the right ear. Now into the forehead.

Exploring now on the sensations in your face. Your eyes, your cheeks, your nose. See if you can feel the temperature of the breath and if that changes when you breathe in and out. Feeling any sensation in your lips, your chin, any tightness in your jaw. Bringing awareness to the very top of the head.

Now, after you have "scanned" the whole body in this way, spend a few minutes being aware of the body as a whole, and of the breath flowing freely in and out of the body.

Now very slowly and gently, while still maintaining an awareness of your body, when you are ready, maybe moving the body a little, wiggling the fingers and toes or gently stretching, then allowing your eyes to open and your awareness to include the room, and the people around you.

Adapted from the Body Scan Meditation, Guided Mindfulness Meditation Practice CDs, Series 1 ©Jon Kabat-Zinn, 2002.

SESSION 1: AUTOMATIC PILOT AND RELAPSE

In this first session, we discuss "automatic pilot," or the tendency to behave mechanically or unconsciously without full awareness of what we're doing. We discuss this specifically in relation to alcohol or drug use (acting upon cravings and urges "automatically" without awareness). We begin this exploration with an exercise called the body scan to practice purposely bringing attention to the body.

SESSION 2: AWARENESS OF TRIGGERS AND CRAVING

This session focuses on learning to experience triggers, cravings, and thoughts of using without automatically reacting. We focus on recognizing triggers and what the reaction feels like in the body, specifically the sensations, thoughts, and emotions that often accompany craving. We begin to use mindfulness to bring greater awareness to this typically automatic process, learning to experience craving and urges in a way that increases our choices in how we respond.

SESSION 3: MINDFULNESS IN DAILY LIFE

We learn the "SOBER space" as a way to expand the quality of mindfulness from formal sitting or lying down practice to the daily situations we encounter. This may help us learn to "be with" various physical sensations and emotions that arise, including those associated with cravings and urges without reacting in harmful ways. In this session, we also begin the practice of formal sitting meditation.

SESSION 4: MINDFULNESS IN HIGH-RISK SITUATIONS

We focus on being present in situations or with people that have previously been associated with substance use, using mindfulness to learn to experience pressures or urges to use without automatically reaching for a substance. We identify individual relapse risks and explore ways to cope with the intensity of feelings that come up in high-risk situations.

(cont.)

SESSION 5: ACCEPTANCE AND SKILLFUL ACTION

It can often feel like a paradox to accept unwanted thoughts, feelings, and sensations. However, this may be the first step in moving toward change. Acceptance of present experience is an important foundation for truly taking care of oneself and seeing more clearly the best action to take. We practice techniques such as the breathing space and focus on using these in challenging situations. This session moves from noticing warning signs and learning to pause to taking skillful action in both high-risk situations and in daily life.

SESSION 6: SEEING THOUGHTS AS THOUGHTS

We further explore awareness of and relationship to thinking, with a focus on experiencing thoughts as merely thoughts (even when they feel like the truth). We look at what role thoughts play in the relapse cycle, specific thoughts that seem especially problematic, and ways to work more skillfully with these.

SESSION 7: SELF-CARE AND LIFESTYLE BALANCE

This session focuses on personal warning signs for relapse and how to best respond when these warning signs arise. This includes discussion of broader lifestyle choices, balance, self-compassion, and the importance of including nourishing activities as part of a full, healthy life.

SESSION 8: SOCIAL SUPPORT AND CONTINUING PRACTICE

In this final session, we review skills and practices learned in this course and discuss the importance of building a support system. We reflect on what we learned from the course and share our individual plans for incorporating mindfulness practice into daily life.

Mindfulness means paying attention
in a particular way:
on purpose,
in the present moment
and nonjudgmentally.

—JON KABAT-ZINN

THEME

Automatic pilot describes our tendency to react without awareness. When we experience cravings and urges to use alcohol or other drugs, we often go into automatic pilot; that is, we act upon them without full awareness of what is happening and what the consequences will be. Mindfulness can help us step out of this automatic pilot mode, helping us raise our awareness and make more conscious choices in how we respond rather than reacting in habitual and self-defeating ways.

HOME PRACTICE FOR THE WEEK FOLLOWING SESSION 1

1. Body Scan

Do your best to practice the body scan on 6 or 7 days between now and when we meet again. There's no "right" way to do this nor is there anything in particular you "should" experience. Just notice whatever is arising in the present moment.

2. Mindfulness of a Daily Activity

Choose an activity that you engage in each day (e.g., washing dishes, drinking coffee or tea) and, as best you can, bring your full attention to the experience in the same way we did with the raisin. You may notice qualities of the object or activity as well as sensations, thoughts, or feelings that arise.

3. Complete Daily Practice Tracking Sheet

Fill this out each day, recording your mindfulness practice (both the body scan and mindfulness of a daily activity). Please be honest. You will not be judged in any way about how much or how little you have been able to practice each week. Note any comments you have about your experience or things that get in the way of practicing.

DAILY PRACTICE TRACKING SHEET
Handout 1.4

Instructions: Each day, record your meditation practice, also noting any barriers, observations, or comments.

Day/ date	Formal practice with CD: How long?	Mindfulness of daily activities	Observations/comments
	____ minutes	What activities?	
	____ minutes	What activities?	
	____ minutes	What activities?	
	____ minutes	What activities?	
	____ minutes	What activities?	
	____ minutes	What activities?	
	____ minutes	What activities?	

Awareness of Triggers and Craving

Between stimulus and response, there is a space. In that space is our power to choose our response. In our response lies our growth and our freedom.
—VIKTOR E. FRANKL

MATERIALS

- ◆ Whiteboard/markers
- ◆ Bell
- ◆ Handout 2.1: Common Challenges in Meditation Practice (and in Our Daily Lives)
- ◆ Handout 2.2: Noticing Triggers Worksheet
- ◆ Handout 2.3: Session 2 Theme and Home Practice: Awareness of Triggers and Craving
- ◆ Handout 2.4: Daily Practice Tracking Sheet

THEME

This session focuses on recognizing triggers and introduces the practice of experiencing them without automatically reacting. We begin by learning to identify triggers and observe how they often lead to a chain of sensations, thoughts, emotions, and behaviors. Mindfulness can bring this process into awareness, disrupting automatic reactive behaviors and allowing greater flexibility and choice.

GOALS

◆ Continue to practice increasing awareness of body sensations.

◆ Practice awareness of physical, emotional, and cognitive reactions to triggers.

◆ Illustrate how these reactions often lead to habitual behaviors and cause us to lose awareness of what is actually happening in the moment.

◆ Introduce mindfulness as a way to create a "pause" in this typically automatic process.

SESSION OUTLINE

◆ Check-In

◆ Body Scan (Practice 1.2)

◆ Home Practice Review and Common Challenges

◆ Walking Down the Street Exercise (Practice 2.1)

◆ Urge Surfing Exercise (Practice 2.2) and Discussion of Craving

◆ Mountain Meditation (Practice 2.3)

◆ Home Practice

◆ Closing

HOME PRACTICE

◆ Body scan

◆ Daily Practice Tracking Sheet

◆ Noticing Triggers Worksheet

◆ Mindfulness of a daily activity

CHECK-IN

Facilitators may wish to review names and/or do a brief one- to two-word check-in ("Name one or two things you notice, or that describe how you are feeling in this moment"). This is best kept brief.

BODY SCAN

Starting in the second week, the first activity of each session is a 20- to 30-minute meditation, followed by a discussion of the experience of the practice. The body scan practice from Session 1 (Practice 1.2) is practiced again in Session 2. Beginning with practice at the start of each session reinforces the experiential nature of the course.

HOME PRACTICE REVIEW AND COMMON CHALLENGES

It can be helpful in this first home practice review to emphasize completion of the worksheets. Working, even briefly, with those who have completed worksheets can reinforce the efforts of these individuals and may provide motivation to those who may not have completed them.

By now, participants have experienced their first week of practicing the body scan meditation at home using the audio recording and have typically already begun to encounter some challenges. Thus, an important objective of Session 2 is to acknowledge and discuss these challenges, address concerns and questions, and clarify misconceptions about meditation. The format and style of this discussion are similar to that described in the previous session, reflecting a sense of curiosity and nonjudgment about the experience of participants. Some of the most common issues that arise in this session are physical discomfort, drowsiness and sleepiness, feelings of restlessness, self-judgment, and expectations about the practice creating a sense of peace and relaxation.

These challenges reflect those described in traditional Buddhist teachings. Although it is not necessary (nor recommended) that facilitators refer to Buddhist terminology in MBRP, this framework can be a useful way to identify the challenges that so often arise for practitioners of mindfulness meditation (Handout 2.1). Traditional mindfulness meditation teachings describe five categories of challenges: (1) "aversion," which could include fear, anger, irritation, resentment, and all of their varied forms; (2) "craving and desire," or the experience of wanting, which may be as subtle as wanting to feel relaxed and peaceful and as extreme as an intense urge to use a substance; (3) "restlessness and agitation," which may be experienced physically, as a strong desire to move, or as mental agitation; (4) "sloth and torpor," which may be in the form of sleepiness, mental sluggishness, or drowsiness; and (5) "doubt," which may be a sense of personal doubt or doubt about the practice and its purpose or utility. A common experience when these states arise is for a meditator to attempt to get rid of them so that he or she can reengage in the meditation, as though these experiences are getting in the way of the practice. Although there are skillful ways to work with these states, observing them *is part of the meditation,* just as observing body states is part of the body scan practice. We are practicing recognition of these states, and cultivating a curious attitude, rather than resisting or attempting to eradicate them. Next we describe some of the common manifestations of these challenges as they arise for participants.

Aversion

The first opportunity to work with the challenge of aversion often arises with the experience of physical discomfort. By the end of this first week of practice, participants may have become more acutely aware of both the sensations of discomfort and pain in the body and their reactions to these sensations. Irritation, self-judgment, and a desire to "fix" or "get rid of" the discomfort are common experiences. Participants may also experience confusion, doubt, and disappointment about the practice based on prior assumptions and expectations about the "pleasant" or "blissful" experiences that accompany meditation. There is often a need for repeated emphasis on the purpose or intention of mindfulness meditation, especially in these beginning sessions. In this second week, we emphasize increasing awareness and acceptance of all phenomena and of one's reactions to these phenomena including uncomfortable or unwanted experiences. We have also found it vital in this session to inquire about some of these experiences, regardless of whether participants voluntarily raise these issues in discussion. Failing to address these experiences increases the risk that participants will become discouraged, feeling as though they are not "getting it" or "doing it right." Fostering a discussion of these common challenges can be especially validating in these early weeks, reflecting the experiences (both pleasant and unpleasant) of all members of the group and emphasizing that no experience is "right" or "better" than any other.

> PARTICIPANT 1: I was really distracted by an itch on my knee and couldn't focus on the instructions. I kept trying to ignore it, but my mind would keep going back to it.
>
> FACILITATOR: What did the itch feel like?
>
> PARTICIPANT 1: It was annoying. I wanted to scratch it.
>
> FACILITATOR: So you noted the itch, then some annoyance, and an urge to scratch the itch. What did the urge feel like?
>
> PARTICIPANT 1: Like restlessness. I felt like it was getting in the way of my doing the exercise.
>
> FACILITATOR: Was there a thought?

PARTICIPANT 1: Yes, I thought, "This is getting in my way. I can't concentrate."

PARTICIPANT 2: I felt the same way about the tension in my back.

FACILITATOR: Okay, thank you. This is a common experience: some discomfort arising, and the desire to make it go away. In your practice this week, you might see what it is like to bring awareness and a sense of curiosity to the itch or the tension. Just noticing, what does an itch really feel like? Is it tingling? Is it hot? Just checking it out, as simply what's arising in the moment. Remember that this practice is about becoming aware of whatever your experience is. Noticing, too, your reaction to it, like the urge to scratch or shift positions, or maybe frustration. What does that feel like? Of course, you can scratch or shift positions if you need to, but just noticing it for a moment before you do that, instead of immediately reacting as we usually do. Why do you think we may want to do that?

PARTICIPANT 3: I don't know. Why would I want to be with pain, especially if I can make it go away?

FACILITATOR: Right, no one wants to feel discomfort. So what might be the value of practicing staying with it?

PARTICIPANT 1: Not just reacting automatically, I guess.

FACILITATOR: So to practice pausing before reacting. How do you think this might be useful in working with relapse?

PARTICIPANT 1: Well, when we have a craving we react just as automatically, without really thinking about it.

FACILITATOR: Yes, we are often not even aware that we are having a craving until it becomes overwhelming or we find ourselves acting on it. Also, craving is sometimes a very physical experience and what we are doing is learning to become more familiar with sensation in our body and what it might be like to just notice discomfort without immediately reacting to it.

PARTICIPANT 2: Avoiding pain is one of my biggest reasons for using. Not just physical pain, but also emotional pain. And look where that got me. The avoiding just doesn't work. Or I guess it works for a brief period, but then it makes it worse.

FACILITATOR: Yes, in a way it gives the pain more power, doesn't it? And sometimes the struggle with the pain is worse than the pain itself. This isn't about punishing ourselves by sitting with pain; it's about bringing gentleness to the pain and struggle, making space for it, so that we have some freedom and we can change our relationship to it in a way that might ease our suffering. When we begin paying closer attention, we may notice there's a difference between the pain itself and our reaction to the pain, like, "I shouldn't be feeling this way." This may make us feel defeated or angry. So we might just continue to practice with these sensations, exploring them a bit. Again, we are being gentle with ourselves here. If you are really stuck or fighting the experience, let it go, change positions, do what you need to do to first ensure that you are taking care of yourself.

Here the facilitator introduces the idea of becoming aware of sensations of discomfort as simply another phenomenon that is occurring in the present moment, and reminds the group that the idea of the practice is not just remaining focused on the breath, to the exclusion of all other experience, but noticing and becoming curious about all phenomena, including discomfort. The facilitator ties this into the experience of craving and our tendency to react automatically. The facilitator also emphasizes that mindfulness is not necessarily about changing one's experience but rather about creating a different relationship to it. This includes creating space for difficult experiences, which may help participants begin to discover that what is so painful is sometimes not the sensation or feeling itself but rather the aversion to it or the ongoing attempts to control our experience.

Craving and Desire

The challenge of craving or desire often arises in the form of a longing for peacefulness and relaxation. It is a common belief among beginning mindfulness practitioners that deep concentration and blissful feelings mean "good" practice and anything less is "bad" practice. However, concentration arises and passes like any other mental state. Yet it's easy for meditators to feel that something is wrong with their meditation when they notice they have been distracted. Many beginning meditators come to the practice with the idea that the purpose is relaxation, and they expect immediate freedom from stress, struggle, and discomfort. They are often disappointed when practice does not always bring about these states. Thus, it is essential to remind participants that we practice to increase our awareness and to develop a spacious, nonjudgmental attitude toward all experience, including discomfort or stress. Experiences of peace or relaxation are thus explored in the same way that discomfort might be, with careful attention to any ideas that these states are the goal of practice.

> PARTICIPANT 1: I found this practice very relaxing.
>
> FACILITATOR: Were there particular sensations you noticed in your body?
>
> PARTICIPANT 1: Just a feeling of ease. I was also less anxious. I noticed my mind wasn't wandering as much. It really worked this time.
>
> FACILITATOR: What do you mean when you say it "worked"?

PARTICIPANT 1: I felt calmer. Usually my mind is just all over the place, and that is one of my biggest triggers for drinking. Just coming back to what is actually going on in the moment. I was really surprised by how well it worked.

FACILITATOR: So you noticed that your mind wasn't wandering quite as much and that you were feeling calmer.

PARTICIPANT 1: Yes.

FACILITATOR: Do you think it will always be relaxing when you meditate?

PARTICIPANT 1: (laughs) No, probably not.

FACILITATOR: So it sounds like a very pleasant experience. And it is also helpful to remember that every time you do it, it is different. Sometimes you might find yourself feeling peaceful and relaxed and experiencing all these pleasant sensations, other times you might feel sleepy or restless or agitated. It is particularly important to remind ourselves that this does not mean that the meditation is "not working" or that we are doing something wrong. It is simply another state of mind to become aware of, just what is arising in the moment. It is very easy to fall into the trap of thinking that the point of practice is to feel a particular way and then to be hard on ourselves if it doesn't meet those expectations. We are practicing becoming aware of everything, all sorts of states, pleasant and unpleasant, to get to know our minds better and to treat all those states with the same interest, curiosity, and openness.

Restlessness and Agitation

Restlessness is a common experience in meditation, experienced both physically and mentally (e.g., racing thoughts, excessive planning or rumination). It is often particularly prevalent in those with higher levels of anxiety and those who are not accustomed to sitting quietly for long periods of time. As with all these challenges, it can be useful to turn one's attention toward the experience rather than attempt to suppress or control it. One might begin by simply acknowledging its presence and approaching it with curiosity, perhaps noticing where it lives in the body and if there is a reaction to the experience.

PARTICIPANT 1: I got tired of the repetition, hearing the same thing over and over again. I noticed that at one point last night I got really agitated. So I just turned it off.

FACILITATOR: What did the agitation feel like?

PARTICIPANT 1: Just restless and like, "When will this end? I just want to turn it off."

FACILITATOR: So it sounds like there were some sensations in the body and the thought "I want to turn this off." If you all remember what we talked about last time: Whatever comes up is part of your mindfulness practice. That includes the agitation, the thought "I want this to end," the urge to act on that thought, all of this. It may be interesting to check that out for a bit: the experience of agitation and the sensations and thoughts that go along with it, noticing any judgment about your experience. Just staying with all of that for even just an extra moment or two.

PARTICIPANT 2: Sometimes when I am practicing, I find that my mind gets caught in thinking about the instructions . . . why is she saying this or that, why is there such a long pause, what's coming next? And then I catch myself and try and come back to the practice.

FACILITATOR: So you noticed the mind getting caught up in questioning or analyzing, and then you guided your attention back. When that happened, was there any judgment?

PARTICIPANT 2: Yeah, like, "Come on, there you go, overanalyzing things again."

FACILITATOR: Okay. Any emotion?

PARTICIPANT 2: Yeah, some frustration.

FACILITATOR: All right, thank you. Again, and we will return to this repeatedly throughout the course, the idea here is not to get rid of the thoughts or even judgment that comes up. We're not fighting or getting rid of anything. We're not even necessarily trying to feel relaxed. We're just pausing and noticing, becoming aware of whatever is going on. So when you find yourself going into analyzing or creating a story about what's happening, the moment you become aware of that, that's a moment of mindfulness. Each time you become aware, simply letting that go and beginning again . . . without forcing or struggling, even if you have to do this over and over again. And if you become aware of struggle, just noticing that with the same gentle attention, letting go of that, starting again.

Drowsiness/Sleepiness

Drowsiness is another common experience in initial meditation practice, particularly in the body scan, which often involves lying down with the eyes closed. This may be in part just the natural response of the body to settling down and taking a break from the hectic pace of our lives. However, sleepiness and drowsiness that occur repeatedly in the course of practice may be viewed as another mental state that can be included in our attention. One might observe the experience of drowsiness itself: What does it feel like? Is it possible to pay attention to the moments when one is startled into wakefulness? What is the mind's reaction to feeling sleepy? Is there self-judgment? If sleepiness is persistent, we might make suggestions for ways to work with this mind state.

PARTICIPANT: I made the mistake of doing it in my bedroom and I fell asleep.

FACILITATOR: What was your response to the sleepiness?

PARTICIPANT: Well, at first, it was fine because it was just relaxing, but when it happened a few times I got a bit frustrated with myself.

FACILITATOR: Were there any physical experiences that went with that frustration?

PARTICIPANT: In my body?

FACILITATOR: Yes, how did you know that you were frustrated?

PARTICIPANT: Just kind of a feeling of agitation and feeling like I'm not listening to the CD.

FACILITATOR: So you felt a physical feeling of agitation and had the thought "I'm not listening to the CD"?

PARTICIPANT: Yeah.

FACILITATOR: So in that moment, you might even bring attention to the experience of frustration, "Hmm. What does frustration feel like?" You might also pay attention to that drowsiness right before you fall asleep, the shift or the startled response when you first wake up, noticing the thoughts that go through your mind and the emotional and physical feeling of frustration. It's possible to make all of that part of your practice; in fact, it *is* your practice in that moment because this is what is happening. We are practicing observing whatever our experience is with curiosity, a more open and relaxed awareness, and without judgment of this experience as "right" or "wrong." Just letting it be what it is.

If you notice sleepiness happening over and over again, though, it might be helpful to sit up straight and be in a more alert posture. You could even practice in a standing posture. You can also keep your eyes open while you are practicing to let some light in, or try practicing at a different time of day. Just experiment with it and see what happens.

Once again, the facilitator draws attention to observing the present moment, including the experience of sleepiness, and encourages curiosity about both its qualities and the mind's reaction to it (e.g., self-judgment, irritation, frustration). She also offers ways to work with it if it repeatedly arises.

Doubt

As stated earlier, doubt may be experienced in several different forms, including doubt about the practice itself or about one's ability to engage in it. Self-judgment is a particularly common manifestation of both aversion and doubt in these beginning stages of meditation. It often accompanies or is experienced as a reaction to one of the other challenges such as sleepiness, restlessness, or discomfort. It may also occur in reaction to a thought, sensation, or emotional state. We have found it useful to repeatedly inquire about experiences of judgment, particularly in response to a challenging or unpleasant arising (e.g., sleepiness, pain, or anger). Inquiring about self-judgment not only encourages greater awareness but presents an opportunity for "letting go," or adopting a wider, gentler, more compassionate stance toward oneself and one's experience. It is also an opportunity for participants to recognize the universality of self-judgment as they hear it reflected in the comments of their fellow group members.

WALKING DOWN THE STREET EXERCISE

The intention of this exercise (Practice 2.1) is to allow participants to observe the initial response of the mind to an ambiguous stimulus and identify the cascade of thoughts, emotions, physical sensations, and urges that follow. The scenario is purposely very simple and intended to be presented briefly. It is important to leave the key stimulus ambiguous; that is, the failure of the imagined person in the scenario to return the wave should be presented with neutral tone and language so the facilitator does not ascribe any meaning to the behavior. This allows the mind to project its own story onto the situation.

Following the exercise, participants are invited to describe any thoughts or images that went through their minds and any feelings, sensations, or urges to react. It may be helpful to list these on the whiteboard. We often use columns to differentiate thoughts, emotions, and physical sensations and to illustrate the ways these experiences affect each other (e.g., a thought eliciting a feeling). As discussed previously, it is sometimes helpful to inquire whether this reaction is familiar, encouraging participants to begin recognizing patterns of thoughts, assumptions, or reactions when encountering triggers or situations that may be unclear or unsettling in some way.

This exercise also allows participants to see the varying interpretations one can make of the same event and to recognize these as "interpretations" or stories rather than "facts." We have found that participants often have difficulty differentiating thoughts from feelings or sensations. Being able to recognize and label one's reactions in this way may help increase awareness of reactions and create a pause in the seemingly automatic chain of experiences. We also use this exercise as preparation for the next exercise, which involves becoming aware of one's thoughts, feelings, and sensations in a situation that is more challenging and may elicit cravings and urges.

FACILITATOR: What did people notice in that exercise?

PARTICIPANT 1: I felt anxious.

FACILITATOR: Okay, and was there a thought associated with that feeling? What happened first, if you recall?

PARTICIPANT 1: First, I felt excited to see him. Then when he didn't wave, I thought, "Why isn't he saying hello to me?" and I felt anxious.

FACILITATOR: So you felt excitement when you first saw him. What did the excitement feel like?

PARTICIPANT 1: Kind of a light feeling, especially in my upper body.

FACILITATOR: Lightness, and then when he didn't wave, you had a thought like "Why isn't he saying hello?," and a feeling of anxiety. Is that right?

PARTICIPANT 1: Yes.

FACILITATOR: So how did you experience the anxiety? Were there thoughts? Sensations in the body?

PARTICIPANT 1: It wasn't physical; it was more mental . . . racing thoughts in my mind and, "Why didn't he wave back? Did he not see me?" or maybe it was personal like maybe I did something.

FACILITATOR: Okay, so that initial thought, followed by more thoughts—maybe stories about why this was happening, trying to make sense of it. And it sounds like there was some self-doubt in there, an assumption that you had done something wrong. Is this reaction familiar?

PARTICIPANT 1: Yeah, it is. I tend to assume that when things go wrong, it's my fault.

FACILITATOR: Okay. Did you notice any urges to react in a certain way?

PARTICIPANT 1: Yeah, I wanted to go home. Isolate.

FACILITATOR: Thank you for sharing that—anyone else have a similar or maybe different experience?

PARTICIPANT 2: I went after him, yelling to get his attention.

FACILITATOR: Okay. Do you remember right before you went after him what you felt or thought?

PARTICIPANT 2: Confusion, then a thought "Did he not see me?" Then this urge to run after him, to fix it.

FACILITATOR: So feeling confusion, then a thought, then an urge. Did you notice any sensations that went along with the urge?

PARTICIPANT 2: I noticed my breathing change. It got a little quicker, sort of more abrupt.

The facilitator might ask for a few more examples using the whiteboard to list thoughts, physical sensations, emotions, and urges in separate columns. This may help participants begin to make these distinctions themselves, teasing apart the seemingly automatic and often overwhelming flood of experience. They may also begin to see how thoughts, feelings, and sensations often proliferate, triggering one another.

FACILITATOR: So you can see here the range of different responses to the same event. Which one is correct? [Participants comment that no one interpretation is "right."] There isn't right or wrong, is there? All just interpretation and reaction. Why might it be important to bring more awareness to these reactions? [The discussion might refer back to the previous week's discussion of stepping out of automatic ways of reacting, giving ourselves more freedom to make purposeful choices.]

When people are asked what they learned from the exercise, they often comment that they recognize how their interpretations of an event affect their thoughts and emotions and how automatic this process often seems. They also begin to recognize how their interpretations may not be reflective of the "truth" and may cause them undue distress or lead to reactive behavior. This exercise lays the foundation for the following exercise in which participants are asked to pay attention to the same type of reactivity in a more challenging situation.

URGE SURFING EXERCISE AND DISCUSSION OF CRAVING

This exercise (Practice 2.2) is designed to shift the relation to experiences of cravings or urges to use substances from one of fear or resistance to that of "being with" in a more curious and kind way. The exercise invites participants to explore a more nuanced experience of craving, observing first the physical sensations as well as the accompanying thoughts and urges, dismantling an often overwhelming experience that might typically elicit reactivity, feelings of defeat or fear, or attempts to control the experience. Participants practice a curious, compassionate presence versus a habitual or automatic reaction. They are invited to look "underneath" or "behind" the craving. Underlying the overwhelming desire for a substance is often a deeper need: perhaps relief from challenging emotions or a desire for joy, peace, or freedom. Recognition of these underlying needs may begin to reveal the deceptive nature of substance use as a refuge and may provide insight into the unmet needs in our lives.

Participants are encouraged to choose a reasonable scenario for this exercise, that is, something that has been challenging or stressful but perhaps not the most challenging situation in their lives or their biggest trigger. They are first asked to picture this challenging situation and then to pause and observe thoughts, feelings, and bodily sensations rather than immediately falling into familiar patterns or reactive behavior. It is suggested that they bring a similar exploration and curiosity to this experience as they did with the raisin or to bodily sensations in the body scan. This exercise is really the core of MBRP; we practice recognizing both the discomfort and the accompanying reactions, including urges to escape it or change an unwanted experience. Then, rather than falling into immediate reaction or resisting the experience, we practice pausing and observing what "craving" actually is. We practice approaching this experience with gentle, nonjudgmental curiosity rather than defaulting to habitual, reactive behaviors.

The "urge surfing" metaphor is introduced in this exercise as a way of staying present with the intensity of craving without becoming subsumed or behaving reactively. Participants are asked to picture the urge as an ocean wave and imagine themselves surfing, using their breath as a surfboard to ride the wave. They ride the wave of craving through its peak and its decline, without being submerged or wiped out by its intensity. We have found that although some participants find this visualization helpful in relating differently to urges, others have difficulty with either visualization or staying present with the intensity of an urge or craving. We have thus presented it as simply one option with which to experiment and have encouraged participants to alter and change the metaphor to suit their individual needs. The primary intention in using the metaphor is to convey the possibility of observing urges and cravings without having to act upon or fight them. This practice not only reveals the impermanent nature of craving, but it also increases participants' confidence in their ability to experience discomfort, and stay present with intensity. We have also found it helpful to highlight how attempts at suppression may be successful in the short term but often result in increased cravings in the long term. This sort of struggle is often unsustainable and ends in a sense of defeat.

We begin by asking what specific physical sensations, thoughts, and emotions arose for people in this scenario. Often craving is accompanied by an emotion, sensation, or thought that feels intolerable and needs "fixing" or from which one desperately needs to escape.

Craving can, at times, be a primarily physiological response to a substance use trigger. However, craving may also mask another emotional state (e.g., loneliness, hurt, resentment, or feelings of betrayal) with an intense desire to alleviate the discomfort. It may also be a sign that our needs are not being met. When cravings arise, it is sometimes helpful to investigate a little further what is really wanted or needed. We find, of course, that it is seldom the thing we are reaching for. The object of desire may be a poor substitute that satisfies us for a moment, but inevitably leaves a deeper dissatisfaction in its wake, intensifying the future cycle of desire.

Following the exercise, facilitators might ask whether participants experienced any emotions or sensations that felt intolerable or urges to escape the experience. Maybe this was accompanied by a thought or belief that they "couldn't stand it" or needed to "fix" it. This can help participants begin to develop a curiosity about their experience, learning to relate to craving differently, perhaps even with curiosity. At this point, however, the main intention of the exercise is to offer an experiential understanding of "being with" the craving rather than "giving in" to it.

Following the exercise, it can be helpful to illustrate on the whiteboard the theory behind urge surfing:

> FACILITATOR: Most of us have the idea that once a craving begins and there is that urge to use, the craving will continue to increase in intensity until we act on it or stop it somehow. We often imagine craving as a straight line continuing upward until we alleviate it by using (*drawing diagonal line sloping upward on the whiteboard*). In reality, craving is less like a line and more like a wave; it ebbs to a peak, and then, if we wait it out, it will naturally subside (*drawing a line increasing, reaching a plateau, then decreasing, like a wave*).

One way to feed the craving is to use a substance in response to it. Using a substance might bring relief. We might feel relief or happiness for awhile, but this is a little like trying to quench thirst by drinking saltwater: You are temporarily relieved, but then you are left even thirstier than you were to begin with. Attempting to fight the craving might be another way to control it. However, when cravings are suppressed, they tend to get stronger. So this is another option: What happens when we just stay right with it?

Each time we practice this surfing, the intensity of the craving tends to decrease a little bit (*drawing shallower curves*), and we get better at waiting it out and become more confident that we are able to ride this wave without getting wiped out.

PARTICIPANT: Maybe that would work to wait it out once, but then the craving just comes back again.

FACILITATOR: Sure, it probably will come back. And if you used alcohol or a drug to make it go away, wouldn't it come back, too? Cravings might arise and pass many times in one day, and this way of being with the experience, or "surfing," may need to be practiced over and over again. It does get a little easier, and the cravings often become less intense because you're not feeding them or fighting them. Whereas when we use in response to the craving we're feeding it, making it stronger, and when we attempt to fight it, we often wear ourselves down and are more likely to feel defeated and want to give up.

There's often the thought or belief "I can't do this." And we're learning that we are able to do this differently, that it just takes practice. You've just done it here; you experienced craving and successfully stayed present without acting on it. Maybe it wasn't as intense as what you might encounter in the future, but just like when you are first learning to surf, you ride small waves first, you practice. Once those become easier, then you can take on bigger ones.

MOUNTAIN MEDITATION

The previous urge surfing exercise may elicit challenging experiences or arousal for some participants. We thus conclude the session with a stabilizing and grounding practice. We have typically used the Mountain Meditation guided practice (Practice 2.3) based on a practice used by Jon Kabat-Zinn (1994). The meditation involves visualizing a mountain and calling to mind qualities of stability, strength, and dignity. Participants are asked to imagine merging with this image of the mountain, embodying these qualities as their own and experiencing a sense of poise and solidity, even in the face of changing circumstances, situations, and inner states. We have found that participants have responded favorably to this metaphor and have little trouble imagining qualities of strength and constancy. However, some participants have expressed discomfort or difficulty imagining themselves as the mountain, either feeling incapable of experiencing such strength and solidity or having trouble with the visualization. Just as with any other practice, we encourage a gentle, kind awareness of the reactions that arise. It may also be useful to play with the metaphor, modifying it as needed. Picturing the mountain is just a vehicle to contact an experience of the qualities it holds, so for those with difficulties visualizing, they might let go of efforts to find an image and invite in the qualities of rootedness, dignity, and strength.

HOME PRACTICE

In addition to continuing daily practice of the body scan and engaging mindfully in a daily activity, participants are asked to use the Noticing Triggers Worksheet (Handout 2.2) to log triggers they encounter over the upcoming week and any subsequent thoughts, emotions, and physical reactions (Handout 2.3). They are also asked to describe any behaviors they engage in to cope with the experience. The purpose of this worksheet is to bring both the triggers and reactions into fuller awareness and to continue the practice of differentiating among thoughts, feelings, and bodily sensations. Participants also complete the Daily Practice Tracking Sheet (Handout 2.4) to supplement their awareness of what they are learning and to give facilitators insight into any concerns or barriers.

CLOSING

Although we have found that typically by the end of the session any anxiety or craving participants experience during the urge surfing exercise has waned, we may invite them to briefly state one to two words to describe how they are feeling after these practices. It can be helpful for facilitators to model this by offering an observation of their own experience (e.g., "peaceful" or "curious").

WALKING DOWN THE STREET EXERCISE
Practice 2.1

Rationale: We are constantly interpreting and judging our experience. These stories and judgments often proliferate, leading to further thoughts, sensations, emotional states, and sometimes urges to react. We might find ourselves in an emotional state or engaging in a behavior with little awareness of how we got there. We would like to use a simple example to illustrate this.

Find a comfortable position in your chair. Allow your eyes to close, if you choose, and take a moment to just settle in. I am going to ask you to imagine a simple scenario and to just notice as much as you can about your thoughts, emotions, and body sensations. Imagine now that you are walking down the street. Picture a familiar location, and really see the sights around you, hear the sounds that might be in this area, maybe cars, birds, people's voices. Or maybe it's very quiet. Now imagine that you see someone you know on the other side of the street, walking in the opposite direction, so the person is coming toward you. Let this be someone you are happy to see—maybe a friend, a co-worker, or anyone who you might want to say hello to. Picture that person now. As you see this person walking toward you, notice what thoughts are going though your mind and any emotions or sensations you may be experiencing.

You smile at this person and you wave. The person does not wave back and continues to just walk by. Notice now what is going through your mind. What thoughts are arising? Notice any feelings or sensations in your body and if they may have changed. Notice if you have an urge to act in a particular way.

When you are ready, allow this scenario to fade, and gently bring your awareness back into the room and open your eyes.

Based on Segal, Williams, and Teasdale (2002).

URGE SURFING EXERCISE
Practice 2.2

Now we are going to do a similar exercise. This exercise may be somewhat more intense than the previous one. We're going to ask you to picture yourself in a situation that you find challenging in your present life, one in which you are triggered in some way, maybe a situation in which you might be tempted to use alcohol or drugs or engage in another behavior that has been problematic for you. Please take care of yourself by choosing something that is challenging but not overwhelming. As you picture this, we are going to ask you to imagine that you do *not* engage in the reactive behavior, whether it is substance use, getting into an argument or fight, or whatever it might be for you. We encourage you to stay with whatever comes up as best you can with a sense of gentleness and curiosity. If the scenario you pick feels overwhelming or like something you do not want to do or are not ready to do, we encourage you to respect that limit. You might imagine a less intense situation in which you react in a way that feels automatic or out of control. For instance, you might call to mind a relationship or a situation where you might react with anger or in a way that's hurtful to you or another person. Do you all have something in mind? If at any point this becomes overwhelming, you can always just open your eyes, maybe move your body around a little bit to reground in the present.

Now I am going to ask you to close your eyes again, if that feels comfortable. You may also leave them open if you choose, maintaining a soft focus a few feet in front of you and letting your eyes just rest there throughout the exercise. Begin by just feeling your body here in the chair. Noticing sensations. Letting the breath flow easily in and out. Now bringing this scenario that you've chosen to mind. A situation that might or has in the past caused craving or urges to act in a reactive manner, in a way that is not in line with how you want to be in your life. Maybe you are with a certain person or in a certain location. Maybe it's something that has happened in the past that you can recall or a situation that you imagine would be challenging for you. Remember that in this scenario you are going to make the choice not to use any drugs or alcohol or to engage in whatever reactive behavior this scenario triggers for you.

Now taking a few moments to really picture yourself in that place or situation or with that person. Imagining the events or situation that lead up to this reactivity, and bringing yourself right to that point where you feel triggered, as though you might behave reactively. And we're just going to pause here for a moment. We often tend to either fall into craving or fight to resist it. Here, we are going to explore our experience a little, finding a balance, just staying with and observing the experience without "automatically" reacting.

So you might begin by noticing any emotions that are arising. Noticing what thoughts might be going through your mind. What physical sensations are you experiencing in this situation? What does this feel like in your body? Noticing, too, what it is about this experience that feels intolerable. Can you stay with it, and be gentle with yourself? If you begin to feel overwhelmed at any point, you can always back off a bit by allowing your eyes to open or letting your attention come back to observing your breathing. Remember that we are practicing staying with this experience in a kind, curious way. We are making the choice to not act on any urges or cravings that are arising . . . just staying with them

(cont.)

and observing, as best you can, what is happening in your body and mind, what a craving or an urge *feels* like. See if you can feel what's here without tightening around it or resisting it.

Feeling what it is like to not engage in the behavior, discovering what happens when you stay with this experience and explore it a little: What is it you are truly needing? Is there a longing for something? Maybe there is fear, anger, loneliness. Maybe relief or freedom. What is it you really need right now? Just staying with this discomfort and unfamiliarity. Observing with a very gentle curiosity.

If a craving or urge becomes increasingly intense, you might imagine it like an ocean wave . . . imagine that you are riding that wave, using your breath as a surfboard to stay steady . . . Your job is to ride the wave of desire from its beginning, as it grows, staying right with it, through the peak of its intensity, keeping your balance while the wave rises, and staying on top of it until it naturally begins to subside. You are riding this wave rather than succumbing to the urge and being wiped out by it. Just watching the pattern as the urge or craving rises and then falls, and trusting that without any action on your part, all the waves of desire, like waves on the ocean, arise and fall, and eventually fade away.

Noticing now how you can simply stay present with this wave instead of immediately reacting to it. Accepting the craving and staying with it, without giving into the urge, without acting on it, without having to make it go away.

Now, taking the time you need, gently letting go of the scenario you've imagined, and slowly and gently bring your attention back into the room. Taking a deep breath if you'd like to. Maybe moving the body a little if that feels right.

MOUNTAIN MEDITATION
Practice 2.3

Settle into a comfortable position, with your spine straight but relaxed, with your head balanced easily on your neck and shoulders, sitting with a sense of dignity and ease. Letting your body support the intention to remain wakeful and present. When you are ready, you might allow your eyes to close if that is comfortable for you. If you choose to keep them open, allowing them to rest in a soft gaze, perhaps a few feet in front of you on the floor. And now allowing your attention to rest on the sensation of the breath as it naturally flows in and out of the body. Just observing your body as it breathes. Coming into stillness, sitting with a sense of completeness, with your posture reflecting this.

Now, when you are ready, bringing to mind the image of a mountain. Picturing the most beautiful mountain you have ever seen or can imagine. Focusing on the image or just the feeling of this mountain in your mind's eye, allowing it to come more clearly into view. Noticing its overall shape: the lofty peak in the sky, the large base rooted on the earth, steep or gently sloping sides. Noticing how massive it is, how unmoving it is, how beautiful both from afar and up close. Its unique shape and form. Perhaps your mountain has snow at the top and trees on the lower slopes. Perhaps it has one prominent peak, perhaps a series of peaks and a high plateau. However it appears, just sitting and breathing with the image of this mountain, observing its qualities.

And when you're ready, seeing if you can bring the mountain into your body so that your body sitting here and the mountain in your mind's eye become one. So that as you sit here, you become the mountain. Your head becomes the lofty peak, your shoulders and arms the sides of the mountain, your buttocks and legs the solid base rooted to your cushion or your chair. Experiencing in your body a sense of uplift from the base of the mountain up through your spine. With each breath, becoming more and more a breathing mountain, unwavering in your stillness, completely what you are, beyond words and thought, a centered, rooted, unmoving presence.

As the sun travels each day across the sky, and light, shadows, and colors are changing virtually moment to moment, the mountain just sits. In the mountain's stillness, night follows day and day follows night, seasons flow into each other, and the weather changes moment by moment, day by day. Calmness abiding all change. In summer there is no snow on the mountain except maybe on the peaks. In the fall, the mountain may wear a coat of brilliant colors. In winter, a blanket of snow or ice. In any season, it may change; it may find itself enshrouded in fog or clouds or pelted by sleeting rain. People may come to see the mountain and be disappointed if they can't see it clearly or they may comment on how beautiful it is. And through all this, seen or unseen, sun or clouds, in sweltering heat or in freezing cold, the mountain just sits. Solid and unwavering. At times visited by violent storms, snow, rain and winds of unthinkable magnitude; through it all the mountain just sits, unmoved by what happens on the surface.

As we sit holding this image in our mind, we can embody the same unwavering stillness and rootedness in the face of everything that changes in our own lives, over seconds, hours, and years. In our meditation practice and in our lives, we experience the constantly changing nature of mind and body, and all the changes in the outer world.

(cont.)

We experience our own periods of light and dark. We experience storms of varying intensity and violence in the outer world and in our minds. We endure periods of darkness and pain as well as moments of joy. Even our appearance changes constantly, like the mountain's, experiencing a weathering of its own.

By becoming the mountain in our meditation, we can touch these qualities of strength and stability, adopting them as our own. We can use its energies to support our efforts to encounter each moment with mindfulness. It may help us to see that our thoughts and feelings, our preoccupations, our emotional storms and crises, all the things that happen to us are much like the weather on the mountain. We tend to take it personally, but like the weather, it is impersonal. In holding it in this way, we come to know a deeper silence and wisdom than we may have thought possible, right here within the storms. Mountains have this to teach us, if we can come to listen.

In the last moments of this meditation, continue to sit with this image of the mountain, embodying its rootedness, stillness, and majesty, until you hear the sound of the bell.

There are some challenges that arise so commonly in the course of meditation practice that the list of these challenges has remained steady over thousands of years. These experiences are not bad or wrong; they are simply part of meditation practice, and they do not mean that your meditation is "not working" or that you are doing the practice incorrectly. These challenges are tricky because when they arise they can be extremely distracting, and people often feel defeated by them. Learning to recognize these experiences as they arise and knowing that they are simply part of the experience of meditation practice can be helpful. It's not just you!

By learning to recognize these challenges in our practice, we can also learn to notice them in our daily lives and notice, too, the ways in which we tend to react to them.

1. AVERSION

This is the experience of "not wanting." Any time we experience something and have the reaction of dislike, or the desire to make that experience go away, it could be described as "aversion." This might include feelings of fear, anger, irritation, disgust, or resentment.

2. CRAVING OR DESIRE

This is the experience of "wanting." It can be as subtle as wanting to feel relaxed and peaceful or as extreme as an intense urge to use a substance.

3. RESTLESSNESS OR AGITATION

This may be a sort of itchy discomfort. It can be experienced physically, as in a strong desire to move during meditation, or as mental agitation, in which the mind feels restless or uncomfortable.

4. SLOTH OR SLEEPINESS

This might be physical drowsiness or mental sluggishness. It might be in the mind, the body, or both.

(cont.)

5. DOUBT

Doubt might be experienced as a sense of personal doubt ("I can't do this practice") or doubt about the practice and its utility ("This is ridiculous. Why would people just sit there and watch their breath?). Doubt is an especially tricky challenge because it can be very convincing. It may help to remember that meditation has been around for thousands of years and has helped millions of people transform their lives. There is no one who cannot participate in meditation; it is accessible to anyone who wishes to practice. It can also be a challenging practice. The important part is to stay with it, and when these challenges arise to bring them, too, into your awareness.

NOTICING TRIGGERS WORKSHEET
Handout 2.2

Pay attention this week to what triggers you to crave alcohol or drugs. Use the following questions to bring awareness to the details of the experience as it is happening.

Day/date	Situation/trigger	What sensations did you experience?	What moods, feelings, or emotions?	What were your thoughts?	What did you do?
Friday 3/26	Example: Had an argument with a friend.	Tightness in chest, cold, clammy palms, heart beating fast.	Anxiety, craving.	I need something to get me through this. How much cash do I have?	Took a walk, later talked with friend about what upset me.

THEME

We tend to either fall into craving or fight hard to resist it. This session focuses on learning to experience triggers and cravings differently. We practice observing the experience without "automatically" reacting. We begin by learning to identify what triggers us, then observing how these triggers lead to all the sensations, thoughts, and emotions that are often part of craving. Mindfulness can help bring this process into our awareness, allowing us to disrupt the "automatic" chain of reactions that often follows a trigger, and giving us greater freedom to make healthier choices.

HOME PRACTICE FOR THE WEEK FOLLOWING SESSION 2

1. Practice the body scan CD on 6 days of the upcoming week, and note your experiences on the Daily Practice Tracking Sheet.

2. Fill out the Noticing Triggers Worksheet each day, noting the thoughts, urges or cravings, emotions (e.g., angry, sad, anxious, happy), and body sensations (e.g., tight in the chest, jittery) you experience. If no triggers or thoughts of using come up on a particular day, you can simply make a note of that. You could also note other types of triggers, for example, things that bring up anger, shame, or any behaviors you would like to change.

3. Continue with the mindfulness of a daily activity practice. You can use the same activity or choose a different one. Bring your full attention to that activity, noticing the sensations, sights, sounds, thoughts, and even emotions that arise.

Instructions: Each day, record your meditation practice, also noting any barriers, observations, or comments.

Day/date	Formal practice with CD: How long?	Mindfulness of daily activities	Observations/comments/ challenges (aversion, craving, sleepiness, restlessness, doubt)
	____ minutes	What activities?	
	____ minutes	What activities?	
	____ minutes	What activities?	
	____ minutes	What activities?	
	____ minutes	What activities?	
	____ minutes	What activities?	

Mindfulness in Daily Life

Drink your tea slowly and reverently, as if it is the axis on which the earth revolves—slowly, evenly, without rushing toward the future. Live the actual moment. Only this moment is life.

THICH NHAT HANH

MATERIALS

- Bell
- Whiteboard/markers
- TV/DVD player
- *Healing from Within* or *Changing from Inside* DVD
- Sitting meditation CD
- Handout 3.1: SOBER Breathing Space
- Handout 3.2: Session 3 Theme and Home Practice: Mindfulness in Daily Life
- Handout 3.3: Daily Practice Tracking Sheet

THEME

Mindfulness meditation can increase our awareness and subsequently help us make better choices in our daily lives. Because breathing is always a present-moment experience, pausing and paying attention to the breath is a way to return to the present moment and bring awareness back to the body. With this presence and awareness, we are often less reactive and can make decisions from a stronger, clearer place. The SOBER breathing space is a practice that can extend this quality of mindfulness from formal sitting or lying-down meditations into the daily situations and challenges we encounter.

GOALS

◆ Introduce formal sitting practice.

◆ Introduce the SOBER breathing space.

◆ Continue practices and discussion of integrating mindfulness into everyday living.

SESSION OUTLINE

◆ Check-In

◆ Awareness of Hearing (Practice 3.1)

◆ Home Practice Review

◆ Breath Meditation (Practice 3.2) and Review

◆ Video

◆ SOBER Breathing Space (Practice 3.3)

◆ Home Practice

◆ Closing

HOME PRACTICE

◆ Sitting meditation, 6 out of 7 days

◆ SOBER breathing space, three times daily (in different types of situations)

CHECK-IN

The check-in is intended to bring attention to a present-moment experience (i.e., "Describe one or two things you notice right now, such as sensations, emotions, or thoughts") or as a time briefly to get in touch with a deeper value or intention (i.e., "What is most important to you to focus on today's session?"). Facilitators can make use of either or both of these practices at the beginning of each session.

AWARENESS OF HEARING

Mindfulness is of limited benefit if it is confined to just the cushion. Although "formal" practices are crucial to building a strong foundation, the real practice is the translation of these perspectives and skills to our day-to-day lives. The importance of this integration is first introduced with the mindfulness of a daily activity exercise in Session 1 and is further emphasized in the present session. Beginning with the awareness of hearing exercise (Practice 3.1), the current session focuses on simple ways to bring attention to activities in which we are constantly engaged but often carry out without awareness. These activities are so automatic for most of us that bringing attention to the actual experience, such as hearing, can be quite an awakening.

This brief meditation has an intention similar to the body scan (i.e., bringing attention to what is already occurring). We are simply exploring this same process through the different senses (i.e., seeing, hearing, smelling, tasting, physical sensation, and consciousness of these experiences).

In group discussions of the hearing exercise in this session and the seeing exercise described in Session 4, we revisit the idea of automatic pilot, returning to the initial intention of stepping out of automatic mode and observing what happens when attention and awareness are brought to any activity, no matter how mundane or routine it might seem. These exercises often illuminate just how automatic the processes of seeing and hearing are, how our minds repeatedly label and categorize these experiences, and how this can obstruct our true vision or raw experience. We have found the seeing/hearing exercises are useful ways to practice direct observation and to begin noticing the mind's tendency to immediately jump in to assess, label, categorize, and judge. Highlighting this tendency of mind in the discussion can be useful.

FACILITATOR: So what did people notice in the awareness of hearing exercise?

PARTICIPANT 1: I heard something moving on that side of the room and thought, "What is that?" Then I really wanted to open my eyes.

FACILITATOR: So hearing a sound, and noticing it was from that side of the room. Then the thought "What is that noise?" and an urge to open your eyes. Anything else?

PARTICIPANT 1: Yeah, I felt like it was cheating.

FACILITATOR: So another thought, "I'm cheating." Some self-judgment?

PARTICIPANT 2: I noticed the pattern of the noise of the traffic outside as the traffic lights changed. I started thinking about how the cars were stopping at the red light, because it would suddenly get quiet. Then there must have been a green light, because the traffic sounds started again.

FACILITATOR: Okay, so first you noticed sounds and the pattern of those sounds, and maybe the mind labeling this as "cars" or "traffic"? Then some thoughts about why the pattern was like that. It sounds like the mind began explaining and maybe even picturing the scene that the pattern was related to.

PARTICIPANT 2: Yeah. At first it was just sound and then I noticed this pattern, and then there was a thought about what was happening out there.

FACILITATOR: The mind wanting to make sense of what you were hearing.

This is something you can try pretty much anywhere, anytime. You can close your eyes or not, depending on the situation, and just listen to the sounds around you, to the textures and patterns. Thoughts will arise about what you're hearing. Just notice that, and see if you can go back to simply hearing sounds as sound, noticing the texture, the loudness, the softness, the pattern of it. There's a tendency to label and analyze it right away, isn't there? So notice that, too.

HOME PRACTICE REVIEW

After 2 weeks of practicing the body scan meditation, participants may have a wider variety of responses and experiences. The body scan practice is intended to help clients raise awareness of what is happening in the present moment in the realm of physical sensation. It is a way to practice paying attention to the body's states and responses from a nonattached, observer's perspective. It may also foster awareness of habits of the mind and barriers to practice. It can be helpful to revisit the Common Challenges in Meditation Practice (Handout 2.1) as examples of aversion, craving, restlessness, sleepiness, or doubt arise.

FACILITATOR: What were people's experiences with the body scan practice this week?

PARTICIPANT 1: It was a lot easier this time.

FACILITATOR: When you say "easier," what did you notice that was different?

PARTICIPANT 1: I did better. I could stay more focused, and could get through the whole thing.

FACILITATOR: So you noticed that you were more able to focus, maybe your mind stayed with the body more and wandered to other thoughts less.

PARTICIPANT 1: Yeah.

FACILITATOR: And it sounds, too, like there's a judgment with that, that this is "good" or "better." Do you remember any thoughts that occurred while you were doing the body scan, about how you were doing?

PARTICIPANT 1: Yeah. (*Laughs.*) I had thoughts like, "Oh, cool, I'm getting better at this."

FACILITATOR: So you're having this experience, a more direct experience, of the body, the sensations, etc. Then a thought comes, evaluating this experience.

PARTICIPANT 1: Yeah. That's what I did.

FACILITATOR: There's nothing wrong here; we're just noticing whatever is happening. Getting to know our minds. Other experiences? How did home practice of the body scan go?

PARTICIPANT 2: I tried to do it. I would keep starting, then would turn off the CD. I just couldn't do it.

FACILITATOR: So what happened? When you say you'd get started and then you'd stop, what happened there when you felt like you needed to stop? Did you notice anything in your body or in your mind?

PARTICIPANT 2: Um, I think . . . I don't know. Like last night, I just wasn't calm enough to sit through it. My mind was scattered, and I wasn't able to really get into it.

FACILITATOR: Okay, this is a really common experience so I'm glad you brought it up. Do you remember the common challenges from last week? Which one might this be?

PARTICIPANT 2: Right—restlessness. I definitely felt that one. Maybe aversion, too.

FACILITATOR: Great. I encourage you to keep approaching it. And notice what is happening as you try it: What does your body feel like? What thoughts are happening? Maybe there's some emotion there, too. Maybe irritation, shame, maybe even anger. So let's see what comes up this week.

I noticed, too, in what you said that there's an assumption that the mind needs to be calm, not scattered, to be able to do this practice. This also comes up a lot. What would happen if you tried staying with it when the mind felt scattered and just noticed what happened?

This happens a lot in practice. We set this time aside and then something gets in the way, either an external distraction like the phone or the kids or something internal like your mind going in 18 different directions, and it's really easy to get frustrated and discouraged. This is something we'll continue to talk about in upcoming weeks, because it will continue to happen. The important part is bringing awareness to what's happening during the practice and in the rest of our lives. So it's okay if distractions happen. Just notice: Recognize that you are distracted, and maybe just check out what *that* feels like. What is my mind doing? What does this feel like in my body? It's another opportunity to pay attention, to observe our experience.

Often in this third week, further barriers and frustrations arise. There is ongoing doubt about doing the practice "right," and questions begin to arise about its purpose.

> PARTICIPANT: I'm practicing what you are trying to teach. This is a new thing and I want to get as much out of it as possible. So I was thinking the other day, how do you incorporate this into . . . I guess I'm not getting it as far as where all this leads to make it something that you would do that would help with urges . . .

> FACILITATOR: Yes, okay. And this is actually the focus of today's session: mindfulness in daily life. How can this foundation that you're building with all of the practices we're doing help you in daily situations? So how might the body scan be used or be useful with urges, cravings, recovery? Do people have ideas? [Here the facilitator is eliciting ideas and experiences from the group rather than "answering" the question.]

> PARTICIPANT: Well, like with the worksheet you gave us last week, I realized I was only putting down emotions and so I started trying to notice the physical reactions I was having, too. I can see how doing the body scan everyday has helped me do that. I don't think I would notice those physical reactions in my body. It's almost like sometimes I don't even have a body. So practicing noticing helps me actually feel what's happening in my body.

> FACILITATOR: Ah, yes. And how might that help with urges or cravings?

> PARTICIPANT: If you can feel where it's coming from in the body you can focus on that part and just relax it a little bit. Slowing down and noticing and taking stock of what's going on instead of just reaching for a drink.

A primary focus of this session is to prepare participants to move into working with high-risk situations by closely observing the reactions that often feel overwhelming and instantaneous. The Noticing Triggers Worksheet (Handout 2.2), assigned in the previous session and part of this week's home practice discussion, is designed to bring the same curiosity to thoughts and emotions that we have been bringing to physical sensations. By bringing attention to what is happening, via any of the senses, we can then begin to observe the associated feelings and reactions that arise around these initial experiences. In discussing the worksheet, we practice again discerning thought, emotion, and physical sensation.

The final column of the Noticing Triggers Worksheet assesses behavior. The purpose of this component is not to evaluate or change the behavior but to begin to expand awareness to include behavioral responses and their consequences. Typically, we do not place a great deal of emphasis on this factor. Sometimes we simply ask, "So you felt angry and a little hurt, your heart was racing, and you noticed some thoughts about how you couldn't go through this again. How did you respond to this experience? What did you choose to do?"

We have found that discussion of the Noticing Triggers Worksheet often elicits storytelling. To continue to maintain a focus on direct experience, we gently redirect participants to the experience rather than the story of the preceding incident. This can be done by explicitly stating that for this exercise we are only interested in participants' direct experiences and their reactions, keeping the description of the trigger to a few words if possible (it is sometimes helpful to ask participants to just read what they wrote on the sheet). Facilitators may need to redirect several times in a session, especially in these beginning weeks.

FACILITATOR: For the discussion of this exercise, I am interested in your reactions and responses more than in the situation that triggered them. Part of what we're doing in here is taking the focus off of that other person, the situation, or the story, and bringing attention to ourselves—to our body, mind, and heart—and how this whole internal system here is responding. So something happened, whatever it was, that triggered you. Tell me, what was the first thing you noticed about your own reaction? Was it physical? A thought? An urge?

PARTICIPANT: I had this experience 3 days ago. I ride the bus a lot and see different areas where people are still using. It takes me to this feeling of being really grateful. And the feeling in my body is like, "Oh, thank God I am not there anymore." At the same time I feel bad for these people.

FACILITATOR: Okay, did you write about this one? Would you be willing to read what you wrote there on your worksheet?

PARTICIPANT: I wrote, "Event: seeing people using on the street. Sensation in body: lonely, sad."

FACILITATOR: So there's emotion—sadness, loneliness. And a memory of yourself out there in the past.

There was an image of yourself out there and some relief that that time is over. You had the thought "Thank God that's not me out there." Then you mentioned, too, feeling sadness and loneliness. Did you notice anything in your body when you felt that sadness and loneliness?

PARTICIPANT: Just a feeling that I don't ever want that to happen again.

FACILITATOR: Okay, so there's a thought, something like "I never want to be out there again." How about physical sensations? Anything you noticed?

PARTICIPANT: Yeah, tightness in my stomach.

FACILITATOR: So it seems like a lot of thoughts about not wanting to be out there, and some memories, maybe, and a lot of emotion—the sadness and loneliness and relief and tightness in your stomach. This is great, that you are noticing all of this.

As in this example, often clients have difficulty discerning a thought from an emotion. In future sessions, we might bring more focus to responses to these initial experiences, such as judgments or frustration for feeling a certain way. In this session, however, the primary focus is on noticing and differentiating between the layers of these initial reactions.

BREATH MEDITATION AND REVIEW

This session introduces participants to the formal sitting practice (Practice 3.2: breath meditation). As practitioners of meditation are aware, posture during sitting meditation can be a helpful reflection and embodiment of the approach to practice. Encouraging and coaching participants to find a posture that supports a relaxed alertness and a sense of self-respect and dignity can support these qualities in the mind. Stiffness can bring about harshness, while laxity can foster sleepiness or fogginess. At this point, many clients still have perceptions of meditation as a "trancelike" state or as a relaxation exercise. It is important to emphasize that these practices are about waking up to our present experience and increasing our awareness, not floating away or escaping. We are practicing staying in this moment rather than habitually calling up the past or inventing a future. Posture can support this intention.

The discussion of this first breath meditation offers an opportunity for facilitators to emphasize once again the intent of this practice; we are simply observing our experience. It is unrealistic to expect that the mind will not wander, when our minds have been "practicing" wandering our entire lives. Beginning the discussion with a question such as, "What did people notice about their minds as they did this exercise?" can encourage discussion of what actually happened rather than what participants believe they were supposed to experience. Bringing some humor and levity here can be helpful; it is difficult to keep the mind on a single focus even for a few seconds!

Because beginning this practice can be so challenging, length of sitting meditations, especially in these beginning weeks, has been the topic of interesting discussions among facilitators of mindfulness-based groups. Colleagues and teachers of related programs have begun the course with brief meditations, lasting perhaps 10 minutes, and likewise suggest 10 minutes of sitting for home practice. Some stay with that period throughout the course, while others describe slowly increasing the time over the 8 weeks to 20 to 30 minutes. We have found with our groups that beginning with the assumption that the participants are able to do the practice, and reinforcing any practice in which they do engage, has led to longer periods of practice than we had initially thought viable. The 30- to 40-minute in-session and home practice meditations allow clients to encounter, and possibly transcend, experiences of physical and affective discomfort. Many participants become most restless after about 15 minutes, and encouraging them to stay with this experience rather than stopping at the peak of their uneasiness allows them to observe this discomfort, refrain from reacting in habitual ways, and to learn new responses.

Although we encourage these sustained periods of meditation, we emphasize that any amount of practice is helpful and reinforce all approaches toward it. We have found that many participants will listen to the whole CD during the first week and continue with the full 45 minutes of daily practice throughout the course, and even beyond the course's end, while others struggle to practice at all. The best approach to home practice continues to be an interesting issue, worthy of further discussion and exploration. We recommend that facilitators follow their own instincts, while being careful not to underestimate or shortchange their participants' willingness or ability.

VIDEO

In this session, as practiced in MBCT, we show a video of other mindfulness-based courses, choosing one that has relevance for the specific group. For example, we have found that certain groups with a history of incarceration respond very well to *Changing from Inside* (Donnenfield, 1998), a documentary that follows a 10-day vipassana meditation course conducted in a Seattle, Washington, jail with individuals incarcerated for drug-related charges. *Healing and the Mind: Vol. 3. Healing from Within* (Moyers, 1993), a video of an MBSR course and one suggested in the MBCT protocol, has also been useful for other groups. Participants seem able to draw parallels between living with chronic pain and living with addiction and with ongoing cravings and urges. The videos often bring an added appreciation and understanding of the process in the absence of seeing others who have been through the course.

SOBER BREATHING SPACE

The formal meditation practices taught in this course are intended to provide the foundation for integrating new perspectives and behaviors into daily life. The SOBER (*Stop, Observe, Breath, Expand, Respond*) breathing space (Practice 3.3 and Handout 3.1) is an adaptation of the 3-minute breathing space used in MBCT. Although we have found the SOBER breathing space to be one of the most useful daily life practices, it is not introduced until Session 3 because of the importance of establishing a foundation of practice to support it. By Session 3, participants have been introduced to the idea of stopping and stepping out of autopilot, and have now had 2 weeks of observing the physical sensations in their bodies, laying the groundwork for the observe step. Similarly, bringing focus to the breath now has a context, and participants have had some familiarity with this practice as well. In a high-risk or stressful situation, a history of meditation can help individuals draw upon these practices. We continue to practice the SOBER mini-meditation in future sessions, presenting it slightly differently each time to continue to generalize the skills.

We have presented the SOBER breathing space from a few different angles. As in MBCT, we often describe it using the image of an hourglass: We begin with a broad focus, then narrow the focus to the breath, and finally expand back out to a wider awareness, illustrating the hourglass, alongside the SOBER acronym, on the whiteboard.

As with many of the practices, there are often expectations for a certain outcome or result. Participants will often comment that it "worked" or "didn't work." Similar to the body scan, sitting meditation, and urge surfing, it is essential to emphasize that the purpose of the exercise is to step out of autopilot and observe; it is to practice noticing, not necessarily to feel differently or to change anything. We often ask what participants noticed, and if there were differences in their experiences during the initial observation and what they noticed when expanding awareness again to the body and mind following the breath focus. It is important to do this carefully, so as not to imply that there *should* be a difference, perhaps even commenting that sometimes there will be and sometimes there won't be, and the important piece is to bring attention to *whatever* is happening.

HOME PRACTICE

In these first several weeks, we encourage participants to spend some time with each of the meditation exercises introduced. Experiencing these different forms of meditation allows a deeper experience of the practice and offers a variety from which participants may choose as they begin to form their individual programs of practice in the final weeks and beyond. Following Session 3, we suggest that participants practice with the sitting meditation audio recordings for 6 out of 7 days of the upcoming week (Handout 3.2). We encourage them to stay with the sitting meditation for the week rather than returning to the body scan, and reiterate that mindfulness includes observation of reactions to the practice (e.g., preference of one over another, resistance or restlessness, or doubt about the practice "working"). We also emphasize that, as with any new skill, the beginning can be frustrating, and it often takes time and effort to learn something new.

The second part of the home practice is to begin using the SOBER breathing space (Handout 3.1) three times daily, both during routine daily activities and in higher stress times. Three times daily may sound overwhelming. However, most of us have been practicing "unawareness" throughout much of our lives. By regularly practicing this technique, we begin integrating it into daily life, replacing the often deeply engrained habit of reactivity with a more mindful response of stopping and observing. We are retraining the mind, and new habits require repetition. If the group seems to be having difficulty completing home practice, facilitators can ask for ideas or creative ways for remembering to use these tools (e.g., while waiting at the bus stop, when getting annoyed with a spouse, or right before eating a meal). Participants are also asked to complete the Daily Practice Tracking Sheet (Handout 3.3).

CLOSING

As in previous sessions, it is helpful to mark the end of the session with a few moments of silence, followed by the sound of a bell, or a brief one- to two-word description of what participants are noticing about their thoughts, feelings, or sensations in the moment.

AWARENESS OF HEARING
Practice 3.1

Take a moment to just get settled in your chair. You can close your eyes or leave them open, however you feel most comfortable. Just allowing yourself to arrive here in the room, feeling your body in the chair, your breath as it enters and leaves the body. Now just letting your attention rest on the experience of hearing, noticing all the sounds. Hearing sounds inside the room and outside it. Hearing sounds both inside and outside of your body. Maybe listening for the quietest sound. As best you can, letting go of ideas or stories about the sounds and just hearing them as patterns, loud or soft, high pitched or low pitched. Hearing the texture of the sounds. You don't need to try to hear anything in particular, just allowing the sounds to come to you, as though you are listening with your whole body, with all of your senses, open and receptive to the experience of sound.

There is no need to analyze or think about the sounds . . . as best you can, just experiencing them. If you find that you are having thoughts such as, "This is weird" or "I don't want to do this" or "I'm not doing this right," simply notice that as well, and gently bring your attention back to the experience of hearing.

Whenever you become aware that you have started to *think* about what is being heard rather than simply experiencing it, gently bring your attention back to simply hearing.

Based on Segal, Williams, and Teasdale (2002).

BREATH MEDITATION
Practice 3.2

Take a moment to settle into a natural, relaxed, and alert posture, with your feet flat on the floor if you are in a chair. It may be helpful to sit away from the back of the chair, so that your spine is self-supporting. How we sit during meditation can be very important. We want a relaxed posture, with our spine straight and shoulders relaxed. The head can be tilted a little forward so the eyes, if open, look down at the floor. Find a posture that embodies dignity and self-sufficiency while still remaining relaxed, not stiff. So take a moment to find that place for yourself, that sense of relaxed alertness. (Facilitators might work with posture here, correcting/suggesting if necessary.)

You may keep your eyes open or closed, whichever feels comfortable to you. Throughout the course, you might want to experiment with both keeping your eyes open and allowing them to close for these exercises. Sometimes it is best to start with eyes closed to better focus your attention on your experience of what's going on in your mind and body. But please do what is most comfortable for you. If you keep your eyes open, let your gaze fall on a spot a few feet in front of you on the floor or on the wall, keeping your focus soft so you are just letting your eyes rest there, not really looking *at* anything.

Now allowing your belly to soften so the breath can flow easily in and out. Softening the muscles in the face, the jaw, the shoulders, and neck.

Letting go as best you can of whatever thoughts or ideas you might have come in with today. Just allowing the past to fall away, and letting go of thinking or worrying about what comes next. Seeing if you can allow yourself for the next little while to just be right here. You might begin by bringing your attention to physical sensations. Bringing awareness to physical sensation can be a helpful way to come into the present, because no matter where the mind is, the body is always present. So maybe now just feeling the weight of your body in the chair or on your cushion. Noticing the places where your body makes contact with the floor and with your chair or cushion. See if you can feel even the light pressure of your clothing against your skin or maybe the air touching your hands or your face.

Now gathering your attention and bringing it to the very next breath. You might feel this in your abdomen as it rises and falls with the inhale and exhale. If it is helpful in focusing your attention, you can put your hand on your belly to help feel the rising and falling. Or you might choose to focus on the area right beneath your nostrils, feeling the air as it enters and leaves the body.

Choose the area where you feel the sensations most strongly and, as best you can, keep your attention there, feeling these sensations of breathing. Follow with your awareness the physical sensations and how they change with each inbreath and outbreath. Seeing if you can notice the slight pauses between the inbreath and the outbreath, and then again the slight pause before the next inbreath.

We are not trying to breathe deeply or change the breathing in any way—simply let your body breathe the way it naturally does. There is no particular way your body is supposed to feel. We're simply observing our body as it breathes, allowing your experience to be just as it is, without judging or needing to change it.

(cont.)

As we sit here with our focus on the breath, the mind will inevitably wander off. This is natural; it is simply what our minds are in the habit of doing. When you become aware that your attention has gotten caught up in a thought or feeling or sensation, simply notice that. You might even gently say to yourself "Not now," and allow your mind to release the thought, bringing attention once again to the very next breath. There is no need to judge yourself when the mind wanders. Simply notice, let go, and begin again with the next breath. This noticing and beginning again is part of the practice.

This may happen a hundred times and that is okay. Simply guide your attention back to the breath, beginning again.

Whenever you find yourself "carried away" from awareness in the moment by thoughts or the intensity of physical sensations, as best you can, bring a gentle, caring curiosity to your experience. Then reconnect with the here and now by bringing your awareness back to the sensations of the breath.

In these last few moments, renewing your intention to stay present, as best you can, beginning again and again, as many times as you need to. Letting go of the thoughts and arriving again right here, with attention on the sensations of breathing.

Now gently expanding your focus to include the room around you and the people here. When you are ready, very slowly and gently allow your eyes to open, staying with this sense of awareness.

SOBER BREATHING SPACE
Practice 3.3

We have been doing a lot of longer meditations, both here and at home. We now want to begin to bring this practice into our lives in a way that can help us cope with daily challenges, stressful situations, triggers, etc. So this is an exercise that you can do almost anywhere, anytime, because it is very brief and quite simple. This is an especially useful exercise when we find ourselves in a stressful or high-risk situation. As we discussed last week, often when we are triggered by things in ourselves or in our environment, we tend to go into automatic pilot, which can result in our behaving in ways that are not in our best interest. This is a technique that can be used to help us step out of that automatic mode and become more aware and mindful of our actions.

1. The first step is to **stop** or **slow down** right where you are, and make the choice to step out of automatic pilot by bringing awareness to this moment.
2. Now just **observe** what is happening in this moment, in your body, your emotions, and your thoughts.
3. Gather your attention and focus simply on the sensations of **breathing.**
4. **Expand** awareness again to include a sense of the whole body and the situation you are in.
5. Now notice that you can **respond** with awareness. We'll talk about this final step a bit more next time.

Let's try this now. You may either close your eyes or keep them open.

1. The first step is to stop, stepping out of automatic mode.
2. The next step is to observe what is happening in your mind and body right now. What is your experience in this moment? What sensations do you notice? Is there any discomfort or tension in your body? What thoughts are present? What emotion might you notice, and where is that in your body? Just acknowledging that this is your experience right now.
3. So now you have a sense of what is going on right now in this moment. Now gathering your attention, focusing attention on the breath, the rise and fall of the abdomen, moment by moment, breath by breath, as best you can.
4. And the next step is to allow your awareness to expand, and include a sense of your entire body. Holding your entire body in this softer, more spacious awareness.
5. Sensing that this is a place from which you might be able to respond to any situation with more awareness.

And then, when you are ready, very gently just allowing your eyes to open.

SOBER BREATHING SPACE
Handout 3.1

This is an exercise that you can do almost anywhere, anytime because it is very brief and quite simple. It can be used in the midst of a high-risk or stressful situation, if you are upset about something, or when you are experiencing urges and cravings to use. It can help you step out of automatic pilot, becoming less reactive and more aware and mindful in your response.

A way to help remember these steps is the acronym SOBER.

S—Stop. When you are in a stressful or risky situation, or even just at random times throughout the day, remember to stop or slow down and check in with what is happening. This is the first step in stepping out of automatic pilot.

O—Observe. Observe the sensations that are happening in your body. Also observe any emotions, moods, or thoughts you are having. Just notice as much as you can about your experience.

B—Breath. Gather your attention and bring it to your breath.

E—Expand your awareness to include the rest of your body, your experience, and to the situation, seeing if you can gently hold it all in awareness.

R—Respond (versus react) mindfully, with awareness of what is truly needed in the situation and how you can best take care of yourself. Whatever is happening in your mind and body, you still have a choice in how you respond.

THEME

Mindfulness meditation can help us increase awareness and subsequently make more skillful choices in our everyday lives. Because breathing is always a present-moment experience, pausing and paying attention to the breath can be a way to return to the present moment and come back into the body. When we are more present, we are often more aware and less reactive and can make decisions from a stronger, clearer place. The SOBER breathing space is a practice that can extend this quality of mindfulness from formal sitting or lying-down practice into the daily situations and challenges we encounter.

HOME PRACTICE FOR WEEK FOLLOWING SESSION 3

1. Practice with the sitting meditation CD 6 days this week and note your reactions on the Daily Practice Tracking Sheet.
2. Begin integrating the SOBER breathing space into your daily life. It is best to practice this in both day-to-day situations as well as in challenging situations. Make a note of your practice on the Daily Practice Tracking Sheet.

Instructions: Each day, record your meditation practice, also noting any barriers, observations, or comments.

Day/date	Formal practice with CD: How long?	SOBER breathing space	Notes/comments
	_____ minutes	How many times? In what situations?	
	_____ minutes	How many times? In what situations?	
	_____ minutes	How many times? In what situations?	
	_____ minutes	How many times? In what situations?	
	_____ minutes	How many times? In what situations?	
	_____ minutes	How many times? In what situations?	
	_____ minutes	How many times? In what situations?	

Mindfulness in High-Risk Situations

When we scratch the wound and give into our addictions we do
not allow the wound to heal. But when we instead experience
the raw quality of the itch or pain of the wound and do not
scratch it, we actually allow the wound to heal. So not giving in
to our addictions is about healing at a very basic level.
   It is about truly nourishing ourselves.

—PEMA CHÖDRÖN

MATERIALS

◆ Bell

◆ Whiteboard/markers

◆ Handout 4.1: Session 4 Theme and Home Practice: Mindfulness in High-
Risk Situations

◆ Handout 4.2: Daily Practice Tracking Sheet

THEME

In this session, we focus on staying present in challenging situations that
have previously been associated with substance use or other reactive behavior. We learn how to relate differently to pressures or urges to use substances,
and practice responding to highly evocative stimuli with awareness rather
than reacting automatically or out of habit.

GOALS

◆ Increase awareness of individual high-risk situations and of the sensations, emotions, and thoughts that tend to arise.

◆ Practice staying with intense or uncomfortable sensations or emotions rather than avoiding or attempting to get rid of them.

◆ Learn skills to help stay present and not automatically give in to pressure to use substances in situations that have previously been associated with use.

◆ Introduce mindful walking as another practice in awareness of various physical sensations and in bringing mindful attention into daily life.

SESSION OUTLINE

◆ Check-In
◆ Awareness of Seeing (Practice 4.1)
◆ Home Practice Review
◆ Sitting Meditation: Sound, Breath, Sensation, Thought (Practice 4.2)
◆ Individual and Common Relapse Risks
◆ SOBER Breathing Space in a Challenging Situation (Practice 4.3)
◆ Walking Meditation (Practice 4.4)
◆ Home Practice
◆ Closing

HOME PRACTICE

◆ Sitting meditation (6 out of 7 days)
◆ Walking meditation or mindful walking, at least two times
◆ SOBER breathing space (daily, especially in challenging situations)

CHECK-IN

Consistent with previous sessions, it is helpful to begin with participants sharing a brief one- to two-word description of their experience. Participants are invited to keep these descriptions focused on present-moment experience and to notice the tendency of the mind to anticipate and prepare a response while awaiting their turn. Facilitators might encourage the group to try *not* preplanning, to listen fully to the others in the group, and notice what arises when their turn comes.

AWARENESS OF SEEING

In the previous session, we introduced exercises to help bring mindfulness from the formal meditations into daily life. This fourth session is designed to continue this integration, with a specific focus on bringing mindfulness into more challenging areas or situations that tend to elicit reactive behavior. Experiential exercises focus on using some of the familiar practices and skills, such as the SOBER breathing space, in the context of a challenging situation. The session begins with a brief exercise in mindful seeing (Practice 4.1). We have found this exercise to be most useful when there is an opportunity to look outside, observing the wind moving through the trees or people or cars passing by. In the absence of a window, we have simply repeated the hearing exercise from the previous session. We are careful to reflect that this exercise is not easy, and that noticing deeply habitual ways in which the mind works (i.e., automatically labeling and categorizing) is part of the practice.

HOME PRACTICE REVIEW

In reviewing experiences with the sitting meditation and SOBER breathing space, it is once again helpful to dispel any expectations of a specific outcome. Participants often have continued expectations about feeling relaxed or having a calm and concentrated mind. Repeatedly reinforcing that the purpose of practice is to become aware of the tendencies of the mind is often necessary, even in this fourth week. In reviewing the sitting meditation, it is helpful to remind participants that observing a wandering or restless mind is part of the practice and an opportunity to observe our reactions to these tendencies.

SITTING MEDITATION:
SOUND, BREATH, SENSATION, THOUGHT

The first sitting practice, introduced in the previous session (Practice 3.2), began with a basic awareness of breath. Each of the following sessions builds upon this practice, expanding the field of awareness to include other sense experiences. The current session's meditation (Practice 4.2) begins again with awareness of sound shifts to awareness of breath, then sensations and thoughts. Future sessions will continue to work with these experiences as well as introduce mindfulness of emotion.

Participants have now worked with the sitting practice for a week and are likely running into both familiar and new challenges. These discussions often allow participants to notice these challenges and share with the group what they have observed over the past week. The content of what comes up is not the focus; it is simply the process of noticing different aspects of their experience, whatever they may be.

PARTICIPANT: The long pauses in the tape drove me crazy.

FACILITATOR: Okay—what did you notice? What was coming up for you during the pauses?

PARTICIPANT: Oh man, I was getting really agitated.

FACILITATOR: Were you noticing that agitation or restlessness at the time?

PARTICIPANT: Oh, yeah. I knew I was agitated.

FACILITATOR: So you noticed agitation. What happened next?

PARTICIPANT: I'd notice it, try to just sort of let it go, or let it be, then try going back to the breathing. I was trying to just sit with it and let the agitation be there, but come back into the moment. Sometimes my mind would immediately go to watching the clock, then the thought "When is this going to end?"

FACILITATOR: Were there sensations, too?

PARTICIPANT: Yeah, my body felt sort of itchy all over, and I just wanted to move.

FACILITATOR: Great. You're noticing agitation, how that feels in the body, then watching how the mind is reacting. Is this feeling of wanting to move or escape familiar?

Often by this point in the course, clients begin to notice changes in their practice and in their responses to what they are experiencing.

PARTICIPANT 1: Early on, I was drifting in and out more noticeably, distracted and hearing other things, but last night, I found my thoughts were pretty much focused on just my breathing, so that was kind of pleasurable.

FACILITATOR: So you're noticing that over this past week, with practice, your mind is able to remain more focused. Was your mind not wandering as much, or were you able to notice the wandering sooner?

PARTICIPANT 1: Kind of both. It was wandering less, and it was easier when I did notice to rein it in.

FACILITATOR: And you said it was pleasurable to have that increased focus. What did you notice about that pleasure?

PARTICIPANT 1: Kind of a relaxation and relief. It feels like it alleviates stress, physical tension.

PARTICIPANT 2: Me, too. It feels like it's getting easier each time, to stay focused on the exercise. I'm still wandering a bit, but I catch myself starting to fade away, then come back. I just started getting an itch when you said to bring awareness to any place of discomfort. So I tried to surround that physical feeling with my focus.

FACILITATOR: What did you notice?

PARTICIPANT 2: I sort of forgot about it.

FACILITATOR: So maybe the first reaction is to scratch.

PARTICIPANT 2: Yeah, almost automatically. I almost reached to scratch it. Then I just stayed with it. Then I went back to the breath, then sort of forgot about it. I don't know, my focus just changed.

PARTICIPANT 3: The more I practice, the more I find that my thoughts do still wander but they tend to come back much more quickly. Early on I had trouble keeping my thoughts from running away, and now it's easier to come back to the moment again.

FACILITATOR: So for you, too, you're noticing that the mind still does its thing, it still wanders off. But you're increasingly able to notice that and to catch it sooner, and to intentionally bring focus back to the present experience.

So we're hearing about some changes that people are noticing. Anyone noticing that their experience is pretty similar to what it was like in Session 1?

PARTICIPANT 3: Well, I find that the breathing just helps me come back. It doesn't really help me from wandering, but focusing on the breath helps me come back. It's the one constant; it's like a home base. That part is easier.

FACILITATOR: Great. I'm glad you are all sharing these experiences. As many of you are describing, and as we have been talking about since the first week, the point is not to keep our minds from wandering. They will wander; it's just what minds do. The idea is to notice, and to practice bringing the attention back, again and again. To realize maybe we have some choice in how we respond to what our minds are doing. And that might get easier with practice. Right now we're just observing our minds, getting to know them a bit better. Seeing what happens when we ask them to focus on a chosen object or experience. And watching how the mind reacts to things that come up while we are doing this.

Often by this fourth week, people begin noticing some changes in how they are responding to these physical, emotional, or cognitive experiences that arise not only in their practice but in how they are responding to daily life situations.

> PARTICIPANT 1: This practice is helping me deal with my wife's drinking. I usually get really upset.
>
> FACILITATOR: What are you noticing that's different?
>
> PARTICIPANT 1: It's helping me focus in on what my emotions are.
>
> FACILITATOR: So in that moment when you're getting upset, what are you noticing?
>
> PARTICIPANT 1: I'm not as quick to act on my anger or judge.
>
> FACILITATOR: So you notice that anger coming up, and then how are you responding to it?
>
> PARTICIPANT 1: What I do now that is kind of surprising is that, instead of yelling, I make sure she is okay and safe, and I feel more compassion.
>
> FACILITATOR: So it sounds like instead of that usual chain of the trigger, then anger, then the familiar reaction of yelling, you are responding differently. Thank you. What are others' experiences?
>
> PARTICIPANT 2: I'm noticing some similar things. It's not anger for me, it's the ability to take a moment and focus on what the real issue might be, what I'm really feeling, how it's affecting me emotionally and in my body. Maybe I am more aware when I start to get caught up in something, then when I start to notice it, I am aware of my mind taking off. Then I just sort of stop and refocus.
>
> FACILITATOR: Yes, and that's the practice right there, to be aware, just noticing that your mind is wandering or "taking off," and maybe stopping right there and intentionally bringing the focus back to the present.

INDIVIDUAL AND COMMON RELAPSE RISKS

One of the primary intentions of this session is to shift from integration of mindfulness into daily life to a specific focus on how these practices might be useful in high-risk situations. Each of us has situations in which we tend to behave reactively, whether it is reaching for a substance, lashing out at someone, or withdrawing. This exercise in identifying high-risk situations not only helps with the recognition of areas that are risky for each individual but highlights reactive patterns common to many of us.

We typically begin by asking participants to share some recent or typical triggers or risky situations. They might refer to the Noticing Triggers Worksheet from Session 2 (Handout 2.2) to identify commonalities in their triggers or just reflect on past lapses or challenging situations. We ask for the general experience or type of situation rather than the story (i.e., conflict with family, situations or settings in which they would use substances, or feelings of anger or loneliness). Writing participants' responses on the whiteboard can be helpful in this exercise. As several examples of challenging situations or triggers are identified, common groupings or categories often emerge. It can be useful to refer at this point to the research on common precipitants of relapse. In the groups we have worked with thus far, the "top three" categories have reliably emerged: negative emotional states ("negative" is traditionally used in the relapse prevention/CBT practice; we often refer to them as "challenging"), social pressure (including social situations associated with substance use that do not necessarily involve direct peer pressure but in which there are felt pressures to use), and interpersonal conflict (often with a family member or partner). Highlighting these categories can bring awareness both to an individual's unique risk patterns and to the commonality of these challenges among all of us.

SOBER BREATHING SPACE IN A CHALLENGING SITUATION

The in-session practice of the SOBER space in a challenging situation (Practice 4.3) allows participants to move from discussion of these situations to direct experience. This exercise allows the experience of pausing right at the brink of where we usually become reactive, breaking the inertia of automatic pilot and bringing awareness to whatever is arising. The exercise is not practiced with the intention to change or "fix" how we are feeling or thinking but to bring greater awareness to the experience just as it is and to allow the space necessary to make a more mindful, intentional choice. This rationale is repeatedly offered to participants and in our experience is never overemphasized.

We might ask participants to pick a recent situation, in which they were triggered or behaved reactively, or an imagined one from the list on the whiteboard. In selecting a scenario with which to practice, we request that people take care of themselves, choosing something that is not going to be too overwhelming or difficult but that provides a sufficient challenge in their lives. Participants often have trouble picking the "right" or "best" scenario. Any situation that elicits a reaction will provide material with which to practice. The situation or feeling that comes to mind first is often a good choice.

In addition to inquiring about the experience after the exercise, it can be helpful to discuss integrating this practice into daily life. For example, what would it be like to do this in a difficult situation? What would make it hard to do this practice in these situations? How might you work with that, or how might you remember to do this practice? In what situations can you imagine this being a useful practice for you?

WALKING MEDITATION

There are several ways to practice walking meditation (Practice 4.4). As with all of the practices, this meditation is best led from experience. The facilitator might narrate the process he or she is engaging in while doing the walking meditation him- or herself. Again, we provide an example at the end of the chapter, but it is our hope that facilitators will not use this as a script, but will lead from their own experience.

Walking meditation can be led as a formal, structured practice ("lifting, placing, shifting") or as a more open awareness of the whole process, allowing a curious, even childlike quality (What is it like to walk? What do the feet feel like as they move? Notice all the muscles it takes to move the leg). The facilitator might offer playful suggestions, such as imagining walking for the first time, as though having just dropped into this human body; and our job is just to observe it as it walks.

Participants might experiment with different speeds. To begin with, one might walk at a pace that is slower than usual, to give oneself a better chance to become fully aware of the sensations of walking. Once participants feel comfortable walking slowly with awareness, they might experiment with walking at faster speeds. If agitation or restlessness arise, it might be helpful to begin walking faster, with awareness, and to slow down naturally as the mind settles.

Walking meditation can be done "formally," in one's home or an appropriate outdoor area, or "informally," outside or in public, in day-to-day life. The practice, similar to a SOBER space, can be a way to check in as one moves through the day. While walking to work or to the bus stop, one might simply note how the body feels, then shift to awareness of sounds, then to the experience of seeing, then to the breath. Or one might simply stay with the physical sensations of walking.

Often people feel awkward, silly, or self-conscious while doing this exercise. Awareness of these reactions, too, is part of the practice. It can be helpful to include all of this when leading the exercise, encouraging participants to notice whatever arises, including any thoughts they are having about the exercise or feelings of embarrassment or silliness, and then focusing again on the experience of walking.

When possible, we lead the group through the initial instructions and then have them move into a larger area to practice on their own for awhile. We encourage participants to pick a short length of ground, and walk the length of that course, turn, and walk back in the opposite direction. The idea is to experience just walking versus trying to get somewhere. In certain settings, it is not possible to walk back and forth or to leave the room to practice, in which case we might stay in the room and walk in a circle.

HOME PRACTICE

Following this fourth week, we ask clients to again practice the sitting meditation or body scan, whichever they choose, for 6 out of 7 days (Handout 4.1). They are asked to practice the walking meditation at least twice and the SOBER breathing space in routine daily experiences and/or when they experience a challenging situation or emotion. Participants are also asked to record their meditation practice using the Daily Practice Tracking Sheet (Handout 4.2).

CLOSING

The session may close with a few moments of silence or with a one- to two-word description of present-moment experience, as done at the beginning of the session.

AWARENESS OF SEEING
Practice 4.1

Sit or stand in a way that you can comfortably see out the window. Take a few moments to look outside, noticing all the different sights. The colors, the different textures, the shapes. For the next few minutes, just see if you can let go of trying to make sense of things in the way that we usually do. Instead, see if you can see them as merely patterns of color, shapes, and movement.

There is no need to analyze or think about what you are seeing . . . as best you can, just experience seeing. If you find that you are having thoughts such as "This is weird" or "I can't do this," simply notice that as well, with gentleness, and bring your attention back to the experience of seeing. Whenever you become aware that you have started to think about what is being seen, or the mind begins telling stories about what you are seeing rather than simply experiencing it, gently notice that and allow your mind to let go of ideas and to arrive again at this experience of simply seeing what is here: the colors, the shapes, lines and edges, movement.

When you are ready, bringing your focus back into the room.

Based on Segal, Williams, and Teasdale (2002).

Settle into a comfortable sitting position. If you are in a chair, place your feet flat on the floor, with your legs uncrossed. Gently close your eyes, or if you choose to leave them open, rest your gaze on a spot a few feet in front of you. Finding your posture, sitting with a sense of dignity, so you are alert and awake and also relaxed.

Feeling the weight of your body in the chair or on your cushion. Noticing the places where your body makes contact with the floor and with your chair.

Maybe taking a moment to remember your intention for being here and committing to being present as best you can for the duration of this practice. Finding that gentle determination to stay with the practice, knowing that you can begin again, refreshing this intention and commitment as often as you need to.

Now just releasing whatever your mind might have come in with tonight. Letting go of the past, of planning or worrying about the future. For now, your job is simply to relax into the present, releasing thoughts as many times as you need to and beginning again with attention to the present experience.

Begin by simply noticing sound and the sensation of hearing. Observing the sounds inside your body and the sounds outside your body. Noticing the texture and the pitch of the sounds. Maybe listening for the quietest or most distant sound. If you find yourself carried away at any time from the experience of hearing, just noting that and gently guiding your attention back to sound.

Now allowing the different sounds to fade into the background of your awareness and resting the attention on the breath, the sensations in your abdomen as the breath moves in and out of your body. Observing the slight stretching as your abdomen rises with each inbreath, and the gentle falling with each outbreath. Focusing your attention gently and firmly on each inbreath and each outbreath. Observing the sensations of the inhale and the exhale, maybe the slight pauses between the inbreath and the outbreath.

There is no need to try to control or change the breathing in any way—simply observe your body breathing. When your attention wants to wander off the breath, just noticing that and gently guiding it back. Letting go and beginning again with your attention resting on the breath.

Now when you're ready, allowing the breath to fade into the background of your experience and bringing your attention to the sensations in the body. Noticing all the different sensations that may be present in this moment, sensations of touch, pressure, tingling, pulsing, itching, or whatever it may be. Spend a few moments exploring these sensations. You might scan the body, from the toes up to the head, or just open awareness to the body as a whole, noticing whatever arises and letting your attention go to that sensation or area.

If you find sensations that are particularly intense, maybe bringing your awareness to these areas and explore with gentleness and curiosity the detailed pattern of sensations there: What do the sensations feel like? Do they vary over time? Continuing to observe the sensations in your body for a few more moments.

When you notice that your awareness is no longer on the body, noting what is on your mind and then gently congratulating yourself; you have already come back and are once more aware of your experience. And beginning again.

(cont.)

Now when you are ready, allowing the sensations in your body to move into the background of your awareness, allowing your attention to move to thoughts. See if you can notice the next thought that arises in the mind. Now watching each thought as it arises and passes away, noticing them as they arise, then gently letting them go. Watching the mind. You might try labeling this process of thinking, simply saying to yourself "thought" or "thinking" as each thought comes. If you notice yourself pulled into a thought or story, just observing that as well and gently letting go, returning your attention again to the awareness of thinking. If you notice your mind repeatedly getting lost in thoughts, you can always reconnect with the here and now by bringing your awareness back to the movements of the breath. Now continuing to practice this on your own for a few more moments.

In the final moments of the meditation, reflecting back on how this practice was for you today. Noticing if there is any judgment about how you did or maybe even who you are. And trusting that anytime we bring mindful attention to our experience, anytime we stop and have the intention of coming into the present, we are nourishing ourselves— taking care of ourselves in a very fundamental way, no matter what comes up during the practice or what our minds and bodies are doing.

Now gently, as you are ready, allowing your awareness to include the room, slowly expanding it to include the people around you. Maybe taking a moment to appreciate yourself and the others here practicing with you. When you are ready, very slowly and gently allowing your eyes to open.

We are going to do an exercise similar to the SOBER breathing space exercise we did last week, taking it a step further. Again, this is an exercise that you can do almost anywhere, anytime because it is very brief and quite simple. It can be used in the midst of a high-risk or stressful situation, if you are upset about something, or when you are experiencing urges and cravings to use.

Can anyone review what the steps are?

Stop and step out of "automatic pilot" in whatever situation you find yourself in. This is the first step in freeing yourself from the automatic pilot mode. Stopping in itself can be a powerful step in making changes in your life.

Observe what is happening right now, in this very moment.

Bring your attention to your breath.

Expand your awareness to include a sense of the body as a whole.

Respond mindfully, with awareness of the array of choices in front of you in this situation. How can you best take care of yourself in this moment?

For this exercise, we're going to ask you to picture yourself in a situation in which you might be tempted to react in a way that is not in your best interest. This might be a situation in which you are tempted to use. But we are going to ask you to imagine, as you did a few weeks ago when we practiced urge surfing, that you do not use or react in any way that is harmful to you or anyone else. We encourage you to stay with whatever comes up with a sense of gentleness and curiosity. If this feels like something you do not want to do or are not ready to do, we encourage you to respect that limit. You might imagine a scenario in which you react in a way that feels automatic or reactive, for instance, a relationship or a situation where you might react with anger or in a way that's hurtful to you or another person. It's best to pick something challenging but not overwhelming.

So let's try this now:

Closing your eyes, if that feels comfortable for you, and bringing to mind a situation or circumstance that has been, or you imagine might be, challenging for you. You might use one we just talked about or think of a different one if you'd rather. This could be a situation or maybe a person or emotion that tends to trigger a reaction in you—maybe craving or urges for substances or maybe an urge to behave reactively. Take a moment to imagine that person, place, situation, or feeling now. Really putting yourself in that story, right at the point where you feel that discomfort or reactivity.

So the first step is to **stop,** right there at that challenging point, and make the choice to step out of automatic pilot.

The next step is to **observe,** becoming really aware of what is happening with you right now, first noticing physical sensations, what is happening in the body. Noticing emotions, now noting any thoughts that might be arising. Noticing, too, any urges you might have to act in a certain way. We're not pushing anything away or forcing anything out, just acknowledge what is happening. Feel what it's like to just observe your experience for a moment.

(cont.)

The third step is to gather our attention in and let it just rest on the **breath,** aware of the movements of the abdomen, the rise and fall of each breath. Just using the anchor of the breath to come into the body and stay present.

Now, having gathered our attention, the next step is to **expand** this awareness to include a sense of the entire body, heart, and mind, including any tightness or tension, emotion, checking in again with the mind and any thoughts or urges. Holding your entire body in this slightly softer, more spacious awareness.

From this place of greater awareness, notice once again the high-risk situation that you are in . . . the situation, the emotion, or the person that is risky for you. And look at the choices you have in front of you. Notice that no matter what thoughts and sensations are going through your mind or body right now, you still have many choices as to how you **respond.** From this place of awareness and compassion for yourself, ask yourself what the best choice is for you, what is most in line with how you want to be in this life, with what is truly important to you. Imagine yourself making that choice, one that leads you away from using or from reacting in any way that is harmful to you or others. As you make this choice, notice again what is happening in your body. What sensations, thoughts, and feelings are here?

When you are ready, gently letting that scene go, allowing your attention to return to this room, allowing your eyes to open.

Adapted from Segal, Williams, and Teasdale (2002). Copyright 2002 by The Guilford Press. Adapted by permission.

WALKING MEDITATION
Practice 4.4

For this exercise we will have our eyes open. Begin by simply standing with your knees soft and arms just resting comfortably at your sides. Letting your focus be soft, maybe just resting on the ground a few feet in front of you. Now bringing your awareness to the bottoms of your feet, sensing the physical sensations of your feet contacting the floor and the weight of your body supported by your legs and feet.

Allow your weight to shift very gently over to the left side, so that the left leg is bearing the weight and the right leg is light. Feeling how the left leg becomes "full" and the right leg sort of empties out. Now shifting the weight back to center, noticing how the body knows where that is. Maybe noticing if there are any urges to shift to the other side. Now allowing the weight to shift to the right, transferring the weight onto the right leg.

Now very slowly taking a step with the left leg, staying with all the sensations as you do this. Feeling the left heel come off the floor, the muscles contracting, the joints moving. Placing that foot down on the floor in front of you and allowing the weight to shift a little onto that foot. Pausing here for a moment. Noticing if there are any urges present—maybe to move the right leg.

And then moving the right leg—lifting the heel and moving the leg forward, placing the heel and then the whole foot on the ground, then shifting the weight forward onto the right leg.

Continuing in this way, lifting the leg, moving it forward, placing it on the ground. Being aware, as best you can, of physical sensations in the feet and legs and of the contact of the feet with the floor. Keeping your gaze directed softly ahead. You might label the movements of each step as a way to focus your attention: "lifting, moving, placing." Or you might allow your attention to move throughout the body as we do in the body scan, noticing all the sensations as you move.

As with the other mediations we have practiced, your attention may wander to thoughts about the exercise or to plans, memories, whatever. When you notice this, just gently let those release and allow the attention to fall back into the present experience of walking.

Now when you are ready, make your way back to your chair, keeping the same quality of awareness as you take your seat.

Based on Segal, Williams, and Teasdale (2002).

THEME

Mindfulness practice can help foster a sense of spaciousness and perspective in challenging situations. In this session, we focus on staying present in situations that have previously triggered substance use or other reactive behaviors. We learn how we might relate differently to pressures or urges to use substances, and practice responding with awareness rather than reacting "automatically" or out of habit.

HOME PRACTICE FOR THE WEEK FOLLOWING SESSION 4

1. Practice sitting meditation 6 out of the 7 days.

2. Practice the SOBER breathing space regularly and whenever you notice challenging emotions, sensations, and urges or anytime you notice yourself becoming reactive. Note your practice on the Daily Practice Tracking Sheet.

3. Practice the walking meditation at least two times this week. The purpose of the walking practice is to connect with awareness of the body while in motion and in day-to-day life. You can practice this formally in a private space, walking back and forth along a short path. You might also practice this in your daily routine, for example, when walking to the bus stop or walking your dog. If practicing in daily life, you may experiment with moving your attention between sensations of walking, the experience of seeing, the experience of hearing, and observation of the breath, resting your awareness on each for a few moments and continuing to move between them.

Instructions: Each day, record your meditation practice, also noting any barriers, observations, or comments.

Day/ date	Formal practice with CD: How long?	SOBER breathing space	Walking	Notes/comments
	____ minutes	How many times? In what situations?	How many times? ____	
	____ minutes	How many times? In what situations?	How many times? ____	
	____ minutes	How many times? In what situations?	How many times? ____	
	____ minutes	How many times? In what situations?	How many times? ____	
	____ minutes	How many times? In what situations?	How many times? ____	
	____ minutes	How many times? In what situations?	How many times? ____	
	____ minutes	How many times? In what situations?	How many times? ____	

Acceptance and Skillful Action

Grant me the serenity
To accept the things I cannot change;
The courage to change the things I can;
And the wisdom to know the difference.
—REINHOLD NIEBUHR

MATERIALS

◆ Bell

◆ Whiteboard/markers

◆ Mindful movement CD

◆ Handout 5.1: Using the SOBER Breathing Space in Challenging Situations Worksheet

◆ Handout 5.2: Mindful Movement Postures

◆ Handout 5.3: Session 5 Theme and Home Practice: Acceptance and Skillful Action

◆ Handout 5.4: Daily Practice Tracking Sheet

THEME

It is important to find the balance between accepting whatever arises while also encouraging healthy or positive action in our lives. For example, we might not have control over things that happen to us, emotions that arise, current job or family situations, or other people's behaviors and reactions.

When we fight against these things, however, we tend to feel frustrated, angry, or defeated, which can be triggers for substance use. When we accept the present as it is, we are not being passive. We are allowing what *already is* without struggle or resistance. This is often a necessary first step toward change. The same is true of self-acceptance; it often requires a complete acceptance of ourselves just as we are before real change can occur.

GOALS

◆ Introduce and cultivate a different relationship toward challenging experiences, such as uncomfortable sensations, emotions, or situations.

◆ Discuss the role of acceptance in the change process.

◆ Introduce mindful movement as another way to practice awareness and acceptance.

SESSION OUTLINE

◆ Check-In

◆ Sitting Meditation: Sound, Breath, Sensation, Thought, Emotion (Practice 5.1)

◆ Practice Review

◆ SOBER Breathing Space (in Pairs) (Practice 5.2)

◆ Using the SOBER Breathing Space in Challenging Situations

◆ Discussion of Acceptance and Skillful Action

◆ Mindful Movement

◆ Home Practice

◆ Closing

HOME PRACTICE

◆ Daily Practice Tracking Sheet

◆ Sitting meditation, mindful movement, or body scan

◆ SOBER breathing space, regularly and when you find yourself in a challenging or high-risk situation

◆ Using the SOBER Breathing Space in Challenging Situations Worksheet

CHECK-IN

Participants may be invited to share one or two words describing their present-moment feelings or sensations.

SITTING MEDITATION:
SOUND, BREATH, SENSATION, THOUGHT, EMOTION

The meditation in Session 5 (Practice 5.1) focuses on awareness of sound, breath, body sensations, thought, and emotion. There is a specific focus on discomfort or any experience that is associated with resistance or tension. This opening meditation lays the foundation for the session's focus on acceptance of all experience, whether pleasant or unpleasant, invited or uninvited.

The use of poetry in meditation instruction and practice has a long and rich tradition. Often poetry can open doors and deepen understanding, complementing the meditation instruction offered by teachers or facilitators. We encourage facilitators to use poetry if and when it feels helpful to the practice.

We sometimes use poetry at the end of the meditation in Session 4, and throughout the course, if and when it feels helpful in conveying the essence of a particular practice. Here we include Rumi's poem "The Guest House," as is often used in MBSR and MBCT, to convey the intention of inviting all experience in as a teacher or guide. Rumi suggests going beyond merely accepting or tolerating challenging experiences, to "greeting them at the door, laughing." Discussion following this meditation might include responses to this (or another) poem and specifically to the idea of appreciatively welcoming all experience, whether it is pleasant, unpleasant, or neutral, because it may provide an opportunity for further discovery and growth.

PRACTICE REVIEW

Participants may notice at this point in the course that they are repeatedly meeting the same challenges and perhaps experiencing doubt regarding whether or not they are "able" to meditate. It can be very useful to review the five common challenges in meditation (restlessness, sleepiness or dullness, craving, aversion, and doubt). We remind participants that these are challenges that have been experienced for thousands of years and are thus very impersonal; these experiences just tend to arise when we ask the mind to maintain awareness, focus, and presence. Facilitators might suggest naming these challenges when they come up in meditation: for example, "Ah, doubt is here" or "This is sleepiness. What does sleepiness feel like?"

Discussion of the SOBER breathing space practice often centers on whether or not participants have remembered and have been able to practice in stressful and/ or nonstressful situations and what they noticed. Again, we often hear comments about this practice "working" or "not working," reflecting the enduring misperception that meditation is supposed to "fix" something. It is helpful to remain aware of this theme and gently bring attention to it when it arises in discussion.

Participants were also asked to practice the walking meditation over the previous week. Again, the focus in this exercise, and thus the discussion, is similar to that of the other practices: bringing attention to the experience, whatever it is, as well as addressing any barriers to practice. People often have experiences with walking meditation that differ from their experiences with sitting meditation. This is neither good nor bad, and simply allows an opportunity to note differences in how the mind responds to the various modes of practice. Issues that sometimes arise with walking meditation are diffusion of focus, feeling "spacey," and feeling embarrassed or silly. Participants are encouraged to notice these experiences, too, as part of the practice. It may be helpful for maintaining focus in walking meditation to return attention to sensations on the bottom of the feet when focus becomes diffuse. Clients might also practice switching from seeing, to hearing, to sensation, and to thought or hold attention on "lifting, moving, and placing" of the feet as a way to focus attention. Participants might play with these different techniques and see what works best for them.

SOBER BREATHING SPACE (IN PAIRS)

The SOBER breathing space (Practice 5.2) is practiced in a somewhat different way in this session. The group breaks off into dyads, and partners are asked to engage in a brief conversation with each other about a typical daily hassle or something that tends to trigger a reaction. We often suggest a topic that most people can relate to, such as transportation issues (e.g., being cut off in traffic, parking hassles, unreliable bus schedules). When it seems as though participants have become sufficiently involved in their conversation, the facilitator rings the bell. Upon hearing the bell, participants are asked to stop wherever they are, even if in midsentence. The facilitator then guides them through a brief SOBER breathing space.

Introducing this interpersonal element, the potential anxiety of having to interact with peers, and the stress associated with daily hassles can help generalize the SOBER practice to a broader class of experiences and contexts. Tension, anxiety, and automatic reactions and behaviors may arise in this exercise, providing an opportunity for participants to observe how rapidly these states can emerge and to practice the SOBER exercise in a slightly more agitated, distracted, or automatic mode.

Discussion of this exercise often centers on noticing experience, with attention to differences before and after the SOBER space. Facilitators may ask about ways in which participants would engage with their partner if they were to return to the conversation following this practice and to notice whether this is different from how they previously have engaged. It can be useful to inquire, too, about how what they experienced in the exercise is similar to or different from ways in which they typically interact in their daily lives.

FACILITATOR: What did people notice?

PARTICIPANT: I noticed that as I was telling my story I was getting back into that same moment again, like I was right back there, and getting upset, and thinking that I shouldn't be upset.

FACILITATOR: So you noticed yourself feeling upset, then the thought "I shouldn't be upset"?

PARTICIPANT: Yeah, that was a thought I had when I heard the bell.

FACILITATOR: What else did you notice?

PARTICIPANT: I was getting heated.

FACILITATOR: Heated—what did you experience?

PARTICIPANT: I was getting angry, getting tense, and I wasn't really breathing.

FACILITATOR: Okay, so when I rang the bell, you noticed anger, some tension and shallow breathing, and the thought "I shouldn't be getting upset."

PARTICIPANT: Yeah. I was like this. (*Tenses body.*) I didn't really notice it while I was talking to my partner here, just when you rang the bell. I sort of dropped in and was like, wow, I am really tense and angry. Then I thought, "Wait, it's over, it's okay."

FACILITATOR: Hmm. Is this familiar at all to you? Do you experience this tension and emotion when relaying a story to someone or maybe just reviewing an event in your mind?

PARTICIPANT: (*Laughs.*) Oh, yeah. I get all worked up over something in my head and I don't even realize it.

FACILITATOR: Okay, thank you. So we see in this exercise how easy it can be to forget these mindfulness skills and get pretty worked up over something that's not even happening. This exercise might be a little closer to how we're usually engaged in day-to-day life and how quickly we lose awareness of our experience. It can be especially challenging to stay present and aware in interpersonal situations, as you might have just experienced.

What is it like, right in the middle of an interaction or experience, to just stop and notice?

USING THE SOBER BREATHING SPACE IN CHALLENGING SITUATIONS

The Using the SOBER Breathing Space in Challenging Situations Worksheet (Handout 5.1) can be introduced following the SOBER breathing space as an extension of this exercise into everyday life. Participants are asked to identify high-risk situations they encounter throughout the week, again differentiating the components of their reactions. The emphasis is on identifying specific experiences, whether physical, emotional, or cognitive, that might serve as cues for practicing the SOBER space. For example, a participant might notice that his breathing changes and his ears begin to feel hot as his anger escalates. These physiological experiences, once identified, might be a useful cue for him to stop and observe his experience. He might bring his focus to his breath for a few moments to gather and ground his attention and then expand awareness to his broader experience and to the situation he is in. Finally, he might respond mindfully, with a greater awareness of his choices in that moment rather than in the habitual manner in which he might typically react.

It is useful to walk through an example in session using the worksheet, identifying specific cues and including ideas of how using the SOBER space might affect the response in a particular situation.

DISCUSSION OF ACCEPTANCE AND SKILLFUL ACTION

Acceptance is at the heart of living mindfully. A fundamental part of the practices included in the course is learning to accept the present moment as it is and to bring attention to our reactions to what has arisen. As we begin to release our struggle with the present moment, meeting it instead with compassion and acceptance, we stop resisting what is true. This letting go can free us from an unwinnable struggle, allowing us greater flexibility and space to see more clearly and to make real changes. We have more freedom to respond instead of react.

As practice becomes deeper and further integrated into our lives, we may begin noticing when we are meeting experience with aversion, attempting to suppress or control what is happening versus acknowledging and allowing an experience, whether or not it is what we wanted. Perhaps we even begin to welcome these challenging experiences with friendliness and curiosity.

The discussion of acceptance and its relation to change often emerges organically at this point in the course. In our experience, the form this discussion has taken has been somewhat different with each group but has centered on the same basic theme. Again, facilitators elicit ideas and themes from the group rather than "teaching" a concept. The following is one example:

FACILITATOR: Up to this point, we have talked a lot about being aware of and accepting physical sensations, thoughts, and emotions, including those that are uncomfortable. We've focused on noticing our experience, and not necessarily *doing* anything, just noticing, raising our awareness of our experience as it is. So where does change fit in? If we just accept everything, how does anything ever change?

PARTICIPANT: Well, you need awareness of what's coming at you, knowing that you can't change a lot of it and so you might as well accept it instead of being miserable and obsessing about it. Because then you just get angry. Like there was this guy who cut in line in front of me at the coffee shop yesterday. I could have gotten really angry and thought about how to get back at him, maybe in the parking lot. I'd get all worked up without even noticing, and what good does that do?

FACILITATOR: So what are you accepting here?

PARTICIPANT: His attitude and that people don't act the way I want them to. That I can't change him, so getting back at him is pointless.

FACILITATOR: How about what's coming up for you in that situation? Does acceptance come in there?

PARTICIPANT: Oh, yeah. I guess I can choose to accept that I am angry, because I just am. But then I can choose how to deal with that, how I want to respond instead of just flying off the handle.

FACILITATOR: This reminds me of the serenity prayer. Who here is familiar with it?

> Grant me the serenity
> To accept the things I cannot change;
> The courage to change the things I can;
> And the wisdom to know the difference.

FACILITATOR: So what are we accepting?

PARTICIPANT: What we can't control.

FACILITATOR: So the acceptance of what is *already here*. What's arrived here in front of us in this moment has already arrived; it's here. We can't change that, can we? It's already happened. That can be a situation, like someone cutting you off in line, or an emotion that comes up, like anger. And we can spend a lot of energy fighting what's already here: "It shouldn't be like this. I hate this. Why is it like this?" or "I shouldn't feel anger." Where does that get us?

PARTICIPANT: It makes us frustrated, angry, stuck.

For many of us, acceptance suggests a passive stance. The intention in this session is to help participants recognize that by meeting an experience with openness and honesty, seeing it as it really is, we are giving ourselves a genuine choice in how we respond. We shift from reacting without awareness or with aversion to responding with a greater sense of space, choice, and compassion. The following is a continuation of the prior dialogue:

FACILITATOR: So this automatic, reactive behavior we've been talking about and working with over the past several weeks often comes from rejection, or nonacceptance, of what is actually happening in this moment. We reject what already *is* because it isn't what we think it *should* be. We are fighting against something we can't change.

We practice this stopping and observing so that we can see this a little more clearly. We accept what is happening in that moment because it is already happening. It's already here. This allows us to start from where we actually are (versus where we wish we were or where we think we should be) and go from there. Does this mean that we can't have goals or work to change things? No, it just allows us to be okay right now, even before we reach a goal or make a change.

PARTICIPANT: First, we have to acknowledge and accept, I guess, what's in front of us. Then we can make a choice about how we want to respond.

FACILITATOR: Yes. A common misconception is that acceptance is passive, that we're letting people or circumstances walk all over us. But we're not talking about accepting being hurt or victimized; it's taking a kinder, gentler attitude toward ourselves and our experience (that's the part we are accepting), so that we can really choose how we act in the world as opposed to just "reacting." This doesn't mean we have to like it. This is about learning to stay with it and make a more intentional choice about where to go from here instead of reacting to it. In a strange way, accepting how things are gives us the ability to change.

The issue of working with anger, whether deep-seated hatred or rage or more subtle forms such as impatience or irritation, often arises as part of the discussion of acceptance and skillful action. Anger can be a powerful emotional state with a decentering quality that can elicit highly reactive behavior. As explored in the previous dialogue, bringing awareness and curiosity to the experience of anger, rather than immediately reacting to it or attempting to suppress it, may help acknowledge its presence and shift attention to the *experience* of the anger rather than to the object of the anger. Bringing attention to the body and physical experience not only may diffuse its charge but often reveals other emotions such as hurt, vulnerability, anxiety, and fear that can underlie the anger. It can be a powerful way to show us the places where we're stuck or hurting. We have found it helpful to include this as part of this session's discussion, using concrete examples of situations that have evoked anger for participants.

MINDFUL MOVEMENT

Mindful movement (Handout 5.2), provides another modality to practice mindful attention. Just as in sitting meditation when we observe sensations of the breath, in mindful movement, we practice paying attention to the sensations in the body while moving, stretching, and engaging in different postures. This is very gentle movement, with a focus on experiencing sensations in the body and tendencies of the mind as we move through different positions.

The presentation and practice of mindful stretching vary with the experience of the facilitators, but it is always important to begin by emphasizing self-care and checking in regarding any physical limitations. Facilitators may choose a few postures that are comfortable for them and suitable for the group. The postures themselves are less important than the quality of attention brought to the practice. Typically, we try a few very simple postures in session, beginning with lying down on the floor, flat on the back, with knees up and feet flat on the floor. We begin very simply with awareness of the body against the floor and of the breath falling in and out of the body. We might move to a gentle arch in the lower back, with hips remaining on the floor, bringing attention to the sensations in the back. Facilitators might move from here into a gentle twist on the floor, dropping knees to one side and turning the head to the other side, to the cat and cow poses on hands and knees or into a child's pose. They might work up to standing, using gentle stretches to the sky, and ending in a simple standing mountain pose or in "corpse" or "resting" pose on the floor, noticing the sensations in the body following the other postures.

As with other practices, this, too, is followed by an opportunity for participants to share their experiences. Facilitators might suggest this practice as another way to become aware of sensations in the body and to practice noticing the wandering mind. Emotional responses may arise as well, because many participants have difficult histories and relationships with their bodies. The practice can also facilitate greater awareness of and a gentle approach to these difficulties, learning to befriend the body, allowing space for emotional and physical discomfort. There may be awareness, too, of the pleasant sensations and the sense of well-being that often arise in mindful movement.

HOME PRACTICE

Following this fifth week, clients are given the choice to practice the sitting meditation, body scan, or mindful movement for 6 out of 7 days (Handout 5.3). They are asked to continue practicing the SOBER breathing space and complete the Using the SOBER Breathing Space in Challenging Situations Worksheet (Handout 5.1). This worksheet helps identify potential cues for taking a SOBER space in situations that might elicit habitual, reactive behaviors. Participants are also asked to record their meditation practice on the Daily Practice Tracking Sheet (Handout 5.4).

CLOSING

As practiced in previous sessions, the session ends with a few moments of silence or sharing a brief description of present-moment experience.

SITTING MEDITATION:
SOUND, BREATH, SENSATION, THOUGHT, EMOTION
Practice 5.1

Take a few minutes now to settle into your chair, finding a posture that feels relaxed, centered, and dignified. Allow your eyes to close if that's comfortable for you. Feeling the weight of your body—where it contacts the chair or your cushion, where your feet or legs contact the ground. The points of contact your body makes with itself—maybe your hands resting on your legs or your arms against your sides. Maybe you can feel the places where your clothing touches your skin.

Now bringing your attention to sounds and the sensation of hearing. You might observe the sounds both inside and outside the body, near and far away. Noticing the texture and the pitch of the sounds. Noticing how the mind labels or makes sense of the sound. Staying as best you can with the raw experience of hearing rather than the thoughts and ideas. As thoughts arise, returning again and again to the experience of sound. And if you find yourself carried away from awareness of hearing, just noting that and gently guiding your attention back to the experience of hearing.

Now letting the different sounds fade into the background of your awareness and allowing your attention to rest naturally on your breath. The inbreath, the slight pause, the outbreath. Aware of the sensations in your abdomen as the breath moves in and out of your body. Noticing that your body knows exactly what to do. Just observing as your body breathes, the slight stretching as your abdomen rises with each inbreath, and the gentle falling with each outbreath. As best you can, staying with each breath as it enters and leaves the body. Each time you notice that your mind has wandered off the breath, gently letting go and beginning again, allowing your attention to return to the breath.

Now when you're ready, allowing the breath to fade into the background of your experience and shifting your attention to the sensations in the body. Noticing all the different sensations that may be present in this moment: sensations of touch, pressure, tingling, pulsing, itching, or whatever it may be. Spending a few moments exploring these sensations.

If there are sensations that are particularly intense or uncomfortable, bringing your awareness to these areas and seeing if you can stay with them, breathing into these areas and exploring with gentleness and curiosity the detailed pattern of sensations: What do these sensations really feel like? Do they change or do they stay the same? Is there a way to experience this discomfort without resisting or fighting it? Noticing any reactions that arise, and meeting whatever is here with kindness. If there is tension, softening those areas as best you can. Seeing now if you can just allow whatever is here to just be.

Now allowing the focus of your attention to shift from sensations to awareness of thoughts. Seeing if you can notice the very next thought that arises in the mind. Then just watching each thought as it appears and passes away. If you notice yourself getting involved or lost in a thought, just observing that as well and gently bringing yourself back to the awareness of thinking. Letting go, beginning again each time you become involved in a thought. If you notice your mind repeatedly getting lost in thoughts you can always reconnect with the here and now by bringing your awareness back to the movements of the breath. Continuing to practice observing thoughts as they arise and pass for a few more moments.

(cont.)

121

Gently shifting your attention now from thoughts to an awareness of any emotions or feelings that might be present. Maybe sadness, frustration, restlessness. Whatever you notice. What is this emotion or feeling? Seeing if you can allow yourself to soften and open to this feeling. What does this emotion feel like? Where is it in the body? Maybe there are specific sensations that go with this emotion. Maybe there is tingling or tension somewhere. Maybe heaviness in the chest or perhaps the heartbeat speeds up. Maybe there is warmth or pressure somewhere. Or maybe it's just a general sense that permeates the whole body. Just see what you can notice. Acknowledging what's there and letting it be.

In these last few moments, seeing if you can hold the whole body in awareness: the breath falling in and out of the body, the other sensations throughout the body, any thoughts that arise.

This is a poem by Rumi called "The Guest House."

THE GUEST HOUSE

This being human is a guest house.
Every morning a new arrival.
A joy, a depression, a meanness,
Some momentary awareness comes
As an unexpected visitor.

Welcome and entertain them all!
Even if they're a crowd of sorrows,
Who violently sweep your house
Empty of its furniture.

Still, treat each guest honorably.
He may be clearing you out
For some new delight.

The dark thought, the shame, the malice.
Meet them at the door laughing,
And invite them in.

Be grateful for whoever comes,
Because each has been sent
As a guide from beyond.
[From Barks (1995). Copyright 1995 by Coleman Barks. Reprinted by permission.]

As the meditation comes to a close, very gently allowing your awareness to expand to the presence of others in the room. Maybe taking a moment to appreciate the commitment and effort involved in engaging in this practice, appreciating yourself and everyone else in this room.

Taking your time—staying with this sense of awareness, spaciousness, and appreciation. Slowly opening your eyes while still maintaining this awareness, allowing your focus to expand out to the rest of the room.

Based on Segal, Williams, and Teasdale (2002).

SOBER BREATHING SPACE (IN PAIRS)
Practice 5.2

We're going to practice the SOBER breathing space, just like the one we did last week, but try it a little differently this time. Once again, you might remember this practice by remembering the acronym SOBER, if that's helpful.

Stop or *Slow* down.

Observe what is happening right now.

Breath focus—centering your attention on the breath.

Expanding awareness to include a sense of the body as a whole.

Responding with full awareness, asking yourself what is needed.

First, we'd like to invite you to break into pairs. Now begin a discussion with your partner about something that frustrates or really annoys you. It could be something that happened today, maybe on your way over here (e.g., maybe someone cut you off in traffic or you spent a long time waiting for the bus). We encourage you to pick something fairly simple, not the greatest annoyance in your life. Does everyone have something in mind? We'll have you talk to each other for a few minutes, then when you hear the bell, stop wherever you are, even if in mid-sentence, and we'll do a SOBER breathing space.

(Allow talking in pairs for a minute or two, then ring the bell.)

Okay, wherever you are, let yourself just stop, right here in this moment. Now observe, just become aware of what is going on right now. What sensations are in the body? What feelings or emotions are present? What thoughts are going through your mind? Just noting the whole experience, without judging it or needing to change anything.

Now gathering awareness by focusing on the breath. By bringing attention to the movements of the rise and fall of the abdomen, to the sensations of the breath moving in and out, and just staying with that for a few breaths.

And now allowing your awareness to expand, to include a sense of the body as a whole, all the sensations that are here. Also an awareness of any feelings or emotions. And checking in, too, on the mind—the quality of the mind and any thoughts that are here.

And then finally, from this place of greater awareness, notice that you can make any one of a series of choices in how to respond. Maybe reflecting briefly on your interaction with your practice partner, and just sensing if there is anything you might want to say or do differently. If you'd like to say anything to your partner, take a moment to do so now. If not, maybe just thank him or her and turn back into the circle.

And then allowing your attention to expand to include the room and gently allowing your eyes to open.

USING THE SOBER BREATHING SPACE IN CHALLENGING SITUATIONS WORKSHEET

Handout 5.1

Instructions: In the left column, list any situations (people, locations, relationships, emotions, events) that happen this week that feel challenging, triggering, or like high-risk situations. In the next columns, write what you notice about your reactions, especially sensations, thoughts, or emotions that might be cues for you in the future to take a SOBER space. In the third column, note whether you were able to take a SOBER breathing space, and in the final column, write your response to this situation.

High-risk situations or triggers (people, locations, emotions, events)	Reactions (sensations, thoughts, feelings that might be cues for taking a SOBER space)	SOBER Space? (yes/ no)	How did you respond?

Notice that the reactions you listed in the second column can be cues for you to **stop** and take a breathing space. See if you can recognize these reactions and begin to use them as a reminder to step out of an automatic, reactive mode and **observe** your experience.

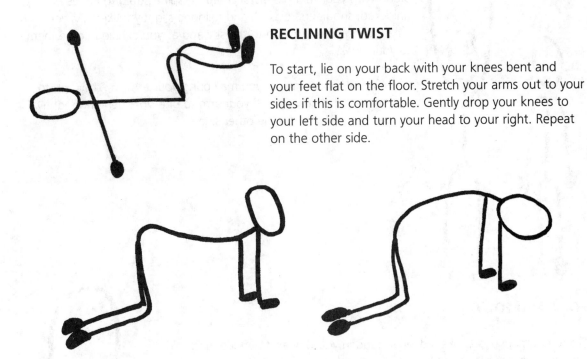

RECLINING TWIST

To start, lie on your back with your knees bent and your feet flat on the floor. Stretch your arms out to your sides if this is comfortable. Gently drop your knees to your left side and turn your head to your right. Repeat on the other side.

CAT-COW POSE

Begin on all fours, placing your wrists directly below your shoulders and your knees under your hips. As you inhale, gently arch the spine, starting from the tailbone and gradually moving up to the neck, turning your gaze toward the sky. As you exhale, round the spine and drop the head, drawing your gaze to your navel. Repeat 10–15 times at your own pace, following the movements of your breath.

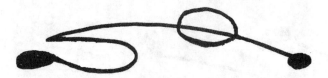

CHILD'S POSE

Following cat-cow pose, allow your knees to drop back to the floor, spreading them wide and letting your belly rest between the thighs. Your arms can either stretch directly in front of you, palms facing down, or can be drawn back alongside your thighs, with the hands facing up. Rest in this pose for several minutes, following the sensations of your breath.

(cont.)

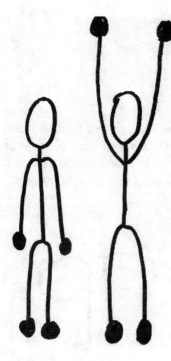

MOUNTAIN POSE

Stand with your feet hip distance apart, spine straight, knees unlocked, shoulders relaxed, and tailbone slightly tucked. As you inhale bring your arms up to the sky and as you exhale release them to your sides.

If you'd like, on an inhale, you may bring your arms up, hold on to one wrist and gently stretch your arm to one side, bending slightly at the waist. Repeat on the other side.

FORWARD FOLD

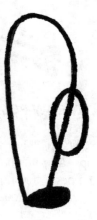

From mountain pose, take a deeper bend in your knees if needed, and fold forward over your legs and letting your hands hang loosely toward the floor or holding on to opposite elbows, just letting the body hang down like a rag doll as you breathe into the back. Feel free to bend your knees as much as you need to. After a few minutes, allow your body to roll up to standing, very slowly, one vertebrae at a time.

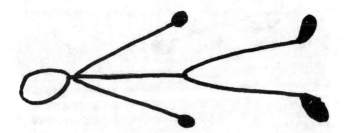

FINAL RESTING POSITION

Complete your movement practice by coming to rest on your back, with your arms alongside, but slightly away from the body, palms facing upward, and the feet falling out to either side. Allow your body to be heavy against the ground and allowing the breath to be natural. Remain in this pose for 5–10 minutes, staying present and aware to the experience of your body and mind.

THEME

It is important and sometimes challenging to accept what is arising in a particular situation. However, this is the first step toward taking healthy or positive action in our lives. For example, we might not have control over things that happen to us, emotions that arise, our current job or family situation, or people's behaviors and reactions toward us. When we fight against these things, however, we tend to feel frustrated, angry, or defeated, which can be triggers for substance use. When we accept the present as it is, we are *not* being passive; we are allowing what already is without struggle or resistance. This is often a necessary first step toward change. The same is true of self-acceptance; it often requires a complete acceptance of ourselves as we are before real change can occur.

HOME PRACTICE FOR THE WEEK FOLLOWING SESSION 5

1. Practice sitting meditation, body scan, or mindful yoga 6 days this week. Note your practice on the Daily Practice Tracking Sheet.
2. Practice the SOBER breathing space regularly and whenever you notice challenging emotions, sensations, or urges or anytime you notice yourself becoming reactive. Note your practice on the Daily Practice Tracking Sheet.
3. Complete the Using the SOBER Breathing Space in Challenging Situations Worksheet.

DAILY PRACTICE TRACKING SHEET
Handout 5.4

Instructions: Each day, record your meditation practice, also noting any barriers, observations, or comments.

Day/date	Formal practice with CD: How long?	SOBER breathing space	Notes/comments
	____ minutes	How many times? In what situations?	
	____ minutes	How many times? In what situations?	
	____ minutes	How many times? In what situations?	
	____ minutes	How many times? In what situations?	
	____ minutes	How many times? In what situations?	
	____ minutes	How many times? In what situations?	
	____ minutes	How many times? In what situations?	

Seeing Thoughts as Thoughts

Our thoughts are just thoughts, not the truth of things,
and certainly not accurate representations of who we are.
In being seen and known, they cannot but self-liberate,
and we are, in that moment, liberated from them.
— JON KABAT-ZINN

MATERIALS

◆ Bell

◆ Whiteboard/markers

◆ Series 2 CDs

◆ Handout 6.1: Relapse Cycle Worksheet

◆ Handout 6.2: Session 6 Theme and Home Practice: Seeing Thoughts as Thoughts

◆ Handout 6.3: Daily Practice Tracking Sheet

THEME

We have had a lot of practice over the past several weeks noticing our minds wandering and labeling what is going on in our minds as "thinking." We have practiced gently returning the focus of attention to the breath or body. Now we want to turn our focus to thoughts, and begin to experience thoughts as just words or images in the mind that we may or may not choose to believe. We will discuss the role of thoughts and believing in thoughts in the relapse cycle.

GOALS

◆ Reduce the degree of identification with our thoughts, and recognize that we don't have to buy into them or try to control them.

◆ Discuss the relapse cycle and the role of thoughts in perpetuating this cycle.

SESSION OUTLINE

◆ Check-In

◆ Sitting Meditation: Thoughts (Practice 6.1)

◆ Home Practice Review

◆ Thoughts and Relapse

◆ Relapse Cycle

◆ SOBER Breathing Space (Practice 6.2)

◆ Preparation for the End of the Course and Home Practice

◆ Closing

HOME PRACTICE

◆ Practice using own selection, 6 out of 7 days

◆ SOBER breathing space, three times daily

CHECK-IN

As an alternative to describing one's experience in the moment, as practiced in the previous sessions, facilitators may begin with a moment of reflection, inviting participants to revisit their intentions for the course and how they wish to integrate the practices learned into their day-to-day lives.

SITTING MEDITATION: THOUGHTS

At this stage in the course, participants have had the experience of using the breath as the primary anchor for their attention, and gradually expanding their awareness to include sounds, sensations, mental states (e.g., agitation, calm, drowsiness), and emotional states (e.g., anger, sadness). Although they have been encouraged throughout the course to become aware of thoughts and the relationship among thoughts, emotions, and sensations, this focus is made more explicit in this session (Practice 6.1). Participants are asked to practice allowing thoughts to be the primary object of their awareness, stepping back from the content of thoughts and observing the nature of thinking itself.

In the current session, we practice acknowledging the presence of "thinking" as yet another phenomenon occurring in the present moment. Through this practice, participants may begin to realize that thoughts are simply words or images arising in the mind rather than reliable reflections of the "truth." Practicing in this way also facilitates the recognition that thoughts need not be the enemy, nor do we have to give them power over our emotions and behaviors. Like sounds or sensations, we can learn to observe them as they arise and pass, while staying in contact with the present moment.

Observing and Labeling Thoughts

In this session's sitting meditation, participants are introduced to metaphors and guided imagery to aid in the practice of bringing awareness to the arising and passing of thoughts in the mind. For instance, they may imagine observing thoughts as leaves floating by on a stream or clouds moving across a clear sky. They are encouraged to experiment with labeling thoughts (e.g., "memory," "fantasy," "analyzing," "planning") to increase recognition of thoughts as passing objects. This practice not only helps to step back from the content of thoughts but allows greater understanding of the various forms thoughts can take.

Following the sitting meditation, participants share their experience and comment on the use of metaphors and labeling as means of observing thoughts. We also suggest a variety of other metaphors, including thoughts as images or words on a movie screen or balloons floating away, and ask participants to be creative in generating metaphors that seem particularly relevant or useful for them. If participants note that their minds are particularly busy, we might suggest metaphors such as listening to a radio broadcast or to a tiny creature on one's shoulder delivering a running commentary; although it may not be possible to turn off the radio or silence the creature, it may be helpful to realize that it is simply a chattering voice and we have a choice in how we relate to it.

The labeling practice may be useful for some in creating distance and perspective. However, for others who do not find it useful or for whom it is a struggle, it need not be practiced. Some participants have had difficulty with the labeling practice and report struggling to find the right label or getting caught up in the labeling itself. The purpose of the exercise is not to focus on the accuracy of the labels but to recognize arising thoughts and the tendency to become involved in them. If finding the "right" label becomes a struggle, a simple label of "thinking" can also be applied.

Often participants will report self-judgment as soon as they become aware of having been caught in a thought or story. This is an opportunity to recognize judgment as yet another thought. Participants are then encouraged to simply note "judging" rather than to try to get rid of judgment, which often just compounds it.

If participants report repeatedly getting lost in the content of a particular thought, they are encouraged to simply return their attention to the breath as a means of stabilizing the mind. Recurring thoughts or themes may reflect a feeling or emotion that one hasn't fully acknowledged or allowed into awareness. If the same thought continues to repeat itself, bringing attention to the feeling state or emotion behind the thought, noticing how it is experienced in the body and mind, can sometimes loosen its grip and power.

On occasion and with continued practice, the mind may be still enough to notice the beginning and end of thoughts and their ephemeral quality, but this recognition takes time and practice. The mind may get caught up in a story for several minutes or even hours before we become aware that we are no longer present. It is unreasonable to expect that our minds will suddenly behave exactly as we tell them to after we have let them run free for so many years. Thus, every moment of awareness and recognition that occurs between these wanderings is a moment of mindfulness and wakefulness; we are simply working to bring into our practice, and into our lives, more of these moments.

HOME PRACTICE REVIEW

In the previous session, participants were given the option of practicing mindful movement in addition or as an alternative to the body scan and sitting meditation practices. Exploring the varied responses to the movement practice is a valuable part of this session's home practice review. Several participants have reported enjoying the opportunity to engage in the practice and relating to their bodies with greater gentleness and caring. This may be particularly helpful for those experiencing significant physical discomfort, stiffness, or pain. Again, it is important to emphasize that the purpose is not to push the body or engage in postures that may be painful but to become aware of the body in movement and to bring care and compassion to experiences of pleasure or discomfort.

Participants sometimes report that the movement practice is easier or more enjoyable than the sitting meditation. In such cases, it is helpful to explore what aspects of the practice are enjoyable as well as those that may be challenging when practicing sitting. Participants may feel that it is easier to be "doing something" rather than simply paying attention to their mental states. In this case, we typically encourage participants to experience each of the different practices with openness, and reiterate that experiences of discomfort, restlessness, or self-judgment that arise are all part of mindfulness practice, allowing valuable opportunities for further observation of the mind.

In the previous session, participants were also asked to continue their practice of the breathing space and to note situations in which they practiced, what they observed, and how they responded. In discussing these experiences, an effort is made to help participants identify specific cues in each of those situations that might be future reminders for taking a breathing space (e.g., shoulders and jaw becoming tense, feeling anger arising, blaming and judging thoughts about my spouse, having the thought, "I can't take this anymore"). Reviewing these aloud can help participants remember them as personal cues for a SOBER space.

THOUGHTS AND RELAPSE

The previous discussion often flows naturally into a conversation about the role of thoughts in the relapse process. We often ask participants to define thoughts, asking whether or not thoughts are "true." This typically leads to the recognition that thoughts are simply ideas, memories, images, and strings of words that arise in the mind from moment to moment that may or may not be reflective of reality. Although some are easy to let go of, others have a more enticing or "sticky" quality.

Participants are often quick to recognize the automaticity of thinking and the link between thoughts and behavior. They typically point out that there is a choice in whether or not to believe, follow, or act upon thoughts. Occasionally, participants have trouble with the idea that thoughts are not always reliable reflections of reality. We have found it helpful to use metaphors and examples to illustrate that thoughts are simply words and images arising in the mind. For example, one might imagine being caught up in the storyline of a movie and having the sudden recognition that one is actually an observer sitting in the audience, that it is only a story. Or one might imagine the mind continually creating thoughts and stories like the heart pumping blood or the stomach secreting bile; it is simply another organ in the body, and producing thoughts and stories is its job. The stories it produces, however, may or may not be grounded in reality. Examples from the group of specific thoughts held strongly to in the past that turned out not to be "true" can also illustrate how untrustworthy our thoughts can be.

RELAPSE CYCLE

To further illustrate the relationship between thoughts and relapse, participants are asked to provide an example of an event that has been or may potentially be a trigger for substance use or relapse. Typically, we choose one example from the group to walk through, illustrating it on the board following the basic template of the relapse cycle (see Figure 6.1). Participants are asked to break down the chain of events by identifying initial thoughts that may have arisen in their minds when encountering the triggering situation as well as any emotional reactions or sensations they may have experienced. They are then asked to follow the situation through to the point of lapse or full-blown relapse or, alternatively, to points in the cycle at which they may have stepped back and responded differently (Handout 6.1). The form that this discussion takes seems to vary from group to group, depending on the unique histories and perspectives of the participants. We have found it most useful to be open to this variability while keeping at the core of the discussion the notion that thoughts play a powerful role at each point in the relapse cycle, and that slowing down and observing one's thoughts, emotional states, and physical reactions can create an opportunity to step out of the cycle and choose a more skillful response. The following is one example of this discussion:

> FACILITATOR: So what is an example of a situation that has led to a relapse in the past or that you imagine could put you at risk for a relapse in the future?
>
> PARTICIPANT 1: Well, say I get into a fight with my wife, and depending on how bad it is it may lead me to want to drink.
>
> FACILITATOR: Okay, so let's just stay with this example and walk through it if that's okay. So the initial trigger is a fight with your wife. What kind of thoughts might come into your mind when that happens?
>
> PARTICIPANT 1: Well, I would be angry.
>
> FACILITATOR: So there is an emotional reaction and probably some physical sensations, too.
>
> PARTICIPANT 1: Yeah, heart racing and blood pressure rising.
>
> FACILITATOR: And what thoughts might you have when you feel this way?
>
> PARTICIPANT 1: Generally, for me it's a "screw it" sort of attitude that leads me to pick up again.
>
> FACILITATOR: So let's break that down. What's a specific thought that might go through your mind?
>
> PARTICIPANT 1: "Screw it, I have been trying really hard and it just doesn't seem to work."

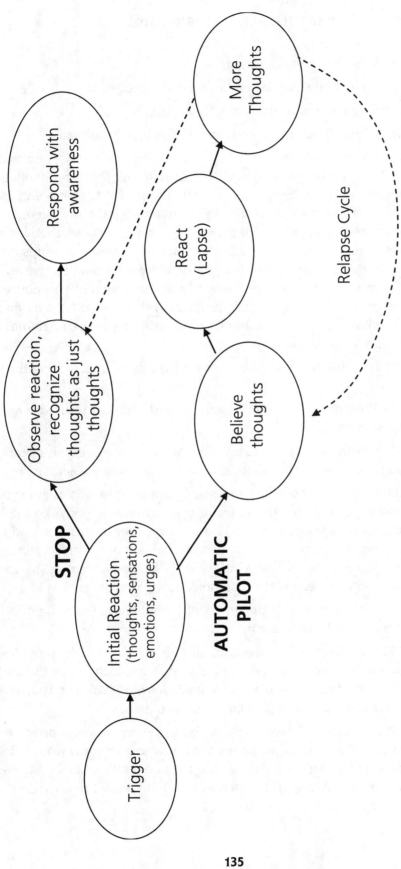

FIGURE 6.1. Relapse cycle. Use the whiteboard to follow a specific example from the group, illustrating the possible paths that different choices will lead to. Highlight the role of thoughts in the relapse process, and the possibility of stepping out of "automatic" and making more conscious choices at any point along the way.

FACILITATOR: What happens after that?

PARTICIPANT 1: I leave the house and head to the liquor store.

FACILITATOR: So it's all really automatic from there.

PARTICIPANT 1: Yeah, I don't stop and observe. It's totally automatic.

FACILITATOR: So another scenario is that you do stop. Let's imagine that for a second. You have the same fight with your wife and the same emotion and the thought, even, of "Screw it, it's not working." Up to that point, maybe none of what has arisen is really in your control—the raw emotion, the physical sensations, and even the thought "screw it." These reactions often just arise when we are triggered; it's what our bodies and minds do and we may or may not be able to change that, at least for now. But we do have a choice in where to go from there. Say at that moment you notice that reaction or that thought, you recognize it, and you stop for a moment to observe what's happening rather than just reacting in your habitual way. What might happen then?

PARTICIPANT 1: I think that would be a powerful way of interrupting this process.

FACILITATOR: What might happen if you stopped and just noticed what you were experiencing?

PARTICIPANT 1: I might realize that my reaction is not necessary; it's irrational. And maybe I would think about the consequences of my actions.

FACILITATOR: Okay, so first of all there is some awareness of what is going on for you—the anger and thoughts of wanting to drink. And you used the word "irrational." Maybe by stopping and noticing how your mind and body are reacting, you aren't believing those thoughts quite as much. Here's this thought, "Screw it, it's not working," and maybe you recognize this as only a thought and notice, too, that you don't have to act on it.

PARTICIPANT 1: If I could stop in that moment, I would have the recognition that it's not true, and I would see that I don't have to go there.

FACILITATOR: So it seems like for you, stopping immediately provides the opportunity to step back and recognize that you don't have to take that route, that you don't have to buy in to what your mind and body are telling you to do. So once you stop, what would you do next?

PARTICIPANT 1: Well, I think I would think about the consequences of my actions and I wouldn't recklessly act on my thought and emotion. I wouldn't leave the house and get in the car to head to the liquor store. Maybe I would go upstairs and be by myself for awhile, or tell my wife I really didn't want to fight anymore.

FACILITATOR: A really different response than the first one.

PARTICIPANT 1: I have gone both ways in this scenario. I've gone to drink, and I've stopped and disengaged from that slippery slope.

FACILITATOR: Okay, then let's follow the other route for a second. Say you do have that thought, "Screw it, not worth it" and you buy into it and drive to the liquor store. What then?

At the final stage in the relapse cycle, participants often have very different reactions to distinguishing an initial lapse from the full-blown cycle of relapse. The discussion follows an example of events and experiences that lead up to a lapse and continues past that lapse to illustrate that, even in the event of lapsing, there is still choice. Reactions to this discussion may vary based on individual histories and experiences. Some participants feel strongly that, after the initial choice of whether to believe the thoughts or after they have behaved reactively to a trigger, they no longer have a choice; it is too late. However, others might consider that the moment of the first drink or use presents another choice point to continue along that path or to stop and turn around. Our approach to this discussion has been to make room for all of these reactions and experiences, while helping participants break down this seemingly automatic process, step by step, suggesting that thoughts following initial substance use (e.g., "I blew it. It's over") are thoughts as well.

The intense self-judgment that often occurs following an initial lapse, referred to as the "abstinence violation effect" (Marlatt & Gordon, 1985), may increase the likelihood of experiencing a full-blown relapse. This discussion can serve as preparation, highlighting the possibility of minimizing the potential damage resulting from a lapse, were it to occur. This discussion also reflects a mindful and accepting stance, encouraging honesty and openness in the face of difficulty. The following is a continuation of the previous dialogue:

PARTICIPANT 1: That's a relapse for me. At that point I am in that spiral and I am not thinking of anything. I'm just on a mission. It's too late.

PARTICIPANT 2: Yeah, me too. If I allow my mind to go from the trigger to following the thought, I am already in trouble. If I don't separate my thoughts at that point, I am a done deal. I am going to end up homeless or in jail and it's all over.

FACILITATOR: So for both of you this is a really crucial point. And yes, it's important to do everything you can to be aware of the direction you're heading in before you end up using. What if we follow this a little further and see what happens? Is it alright if we do that? In the past, when you have gotten to the point of using and spiraled so quickly, is there anything you can think of that might have helped you turn around a little sooner? That might have prevented you from going so far down that path until you ended up homeless or in jail?

[Facilitator and participant review the thoughts and actions in this participant's familiar scenario, pausing at each step to recognize what thoughts might have been arising, whether or not those thoughts were "trustworthy" or "true," and the effects of believing those thoughts. The facilitator also highlights all the cues the participant might notice in the future for taking a SOBER space and stepping out of the cycle, even when his mind was telling him it was "too late."]

FACILITATOR: It's going to be a different process for each person. What's important is that you get to know how your mind works, and points at which you've gotten in trouble in the past where maybe you could do something differently if that were to come up again. What we are doing here is highlighting different points at which you may have a choice and can shift the course. So, in this example, when you get to this point here (where you have had the first drink), what goes through your mind?

PARTICIPANT 3: I've already screwed up.

FACILITATOR: Right, "I've already screwed up, why stop now? I might as well go all the way."

PARTICIPANT 3: Exactly.

FACILITATOR: And even though you are already in trouble at this point, does it have to be all over? That thought, "I've already screwed up," even though it is an extremely powerful and consuming thought, it is still a thought. I don't want to minimize the dangerousness and seriousness of the situation, but if you do end up in this very dangerous place, does it have to be "a done deal"?

PARTICIPANT 3: No.

FACILITATOR: It might feel like it's all over, but in reality you still have a choice, even at this point. Every time we talk about this, people have very different reactions, and with good reason. It's a scary and dangerous place to be. We're getting a better understanding of how our minds behave in these situations, seeing the different points in the process where we get stuck, and seeing different points where we may be able to stop and do something differently. The sooner the better, but if we do get this far, there are things we can do to turn around, to decrease the damage. The idea in talking through this is not that you shouldn't do everything in your power to not end up in this place. It's like practicing a fire drill; it certainly doesn't mean that you have to go set a fire! We do everything we can to prevent a fire from starting, because it's not what we want. But if it does happen, we want to be prepared so we can get out safely and minimize the damage.

SOBER BREATHING SPACE

Given that participants often have strong reactions to this conversation, it can be helpful to conclude with a SOBER breathing space (Practice 6.2) as an opportunity to observe one's reactions, thoughts, and emotions and to reconnect with the present. The SOBER breathing space in this session might emphasize a focus on arising thoughts.

PREPARATION FOR THE END OF THE COURSE AND HOME PRACTICE

At this stage in the program, participants are encouraged to begin exploring ways to personalize the practice and make it a part of their daily lives. In this spirit, they are encouraged to choose a selection of practices from the options offered in the previous weeks (Handout 6.2). It can be helpful to provide additional audio recordings of shorter practices of 10, 20, and 30 minutes or practices without verbal instructions (just the sound of a bell as a reminder to return awareness to the present). Although participants may experiment with combinations of these practices, they are encouraged to continue with a total of 40 minutes of practice per day to maintain and continue to build on the skills gained during the course. In preparation for continuing practice following the course, participants are asked to begin reflecting on what they have learned over the past several weeks and which practices they intend to continue. It is suggested that they continue practicing the SOBER breathing space as part of their daily lives, particularly in situations where they find themselves overwhelmed or reactive. Participants are also asked to record their meditation practice on the Daily Practice Tracking Sheet (Handout 6.3).

CLOSING

Facilitators may choose to close with a moment of silence or a brief checkout.

SITTING MEDITATION: THOUGHTS
Practice 6.1

Begin by settling in your chair, closing your eyes if you choose to. Sitting with a calm, dignified, and wakeful presence, with your spine straight and body relaxed. Take a moment to let yourself become aware of yourself here in this room at this moment. Allowing awareness of your body here in the chair.

Now gathering the attention and bringing it to your breath: the inbreath, the outbreath, the waves of breath as they enter and leave your body. Not looking for anything to happen or for any special state or experience, just continuing to stay with the sensations of breathing for the next few moments.

Now letting the breath fade into the background, allowing your awareness to focus on the thoughts that arise in your mind. See if you can just notice the very next thought that arises in your mind, and letting it naturally pass by, and the next thought, allowing that to pass by, too, without becoming involved in it or following it.

You might imagine that you are sitting by a stream. Take a moment now to picture this stream in your mind. Now, as thoughts begin to arise, imagine you are sitting on the shore, watching them float by as though they were leaves on the water. As you become aware of each thought that appears, just gently allow it to float by. The thoughts might be words or an image or a sentence. Some thoughts might be larger or heavier, some smaller, quicker, or lighter. Whatever form the thought is in, as the next one appears, do the same—allowing it to float by. Just doing your best with this. If you find that you are worrying about what it should look like or whether you are doing this right, just notice that these, too, are thoughts on the passing stream. If thoughts come quickly, you might picture the stream rushing with white water. As the thoughts calm down, the stream might slow down and flow more smoothly.

If you find that you become lost in a thought or your attention has wandered, you might congratulate yourself for becoming aware again, noticing, if possible, what thought pulled you away and then simply beginning again, bringing your awareness back to observing your thoughts.

If you find yourself following the thoughts, as often happens, as soon as you notice that they have carried you away from the present, simply stepping out of the stream brings your attention back to sitting on the bank observing.

Something you might try here is labeling thoughts as they appear. Maybe they are judgments about yourself, your experience, or of how you are doing in this exercise. If so, just label that thought as "judgment" and let it pass. Perhaps you have a memory arise. If so, you might just label it as "memory." Or perhaps plans come to mind about what you are going to do after today's session or what you are going to say to someone in the future. Often fantasies come to mind. We imagine scenarios that might happen or that we would like to happen. Just recognize the thoughts as judgments, memories, plans, fantasies, or any labels that work for you, and allow the thoughts to pass. Try practicing this now. If no labels come to mind, that's okay, too. You might just use the label "thought" or simply notice that no labels come to mind and continue to observe.

(cont.)

If you find you are lost in one of the thoughts that has arisen, notice what that thought was that carried you away, then gently bring yourself back to the exercise of observing.

Now, very gently and when you are ready, allowing your awareness to focus on the room here, your body in this chair, awareness of the other people here with you in the room. Giving yourself time to very gently allow your eyes to open. Holding this awareness, as best you can, as your eyes take in the room and the people around you.

SOBER BREATHING SPACE
Practice 6.2

Let's take a moment to stop right here. Begin by just observing, becoming aware, really aware, of what is going on with you right now—sensations, emotions, and thoughts. Pay particular attention this time to what thoughts are arising. What are you saying to yourself? What is the quality of your mind right now? Is it calm? Agitated? Rushing with thoughts?

Now bringing awareness to the breath . . . the movements of the abdomen, the rise and fall of the breath, moment by moment, breath by breath.

Now allowing our awareness to expand to include a sense of the body as a whole. Following the breath as if your whole body is breathing. Holding your entire body in this slightly softer, more spacious awareness, noticing again the thoughts that are present. Noticing the quality of the mind.

Adapted from Segal, Williams, and Teasdale (2002). Copyright 2002 by The Guilford Press. Adapted by permission.

RELAPSE CYCLE WORKSHEET
Handout 6.1

Think of a situation that has led to relapse in the past or a situation you imagine might be risky for you. Write the trigger, the initial reaction that followed, and the events along each possible path in the circles below. *What are the different ways that you might respond?*

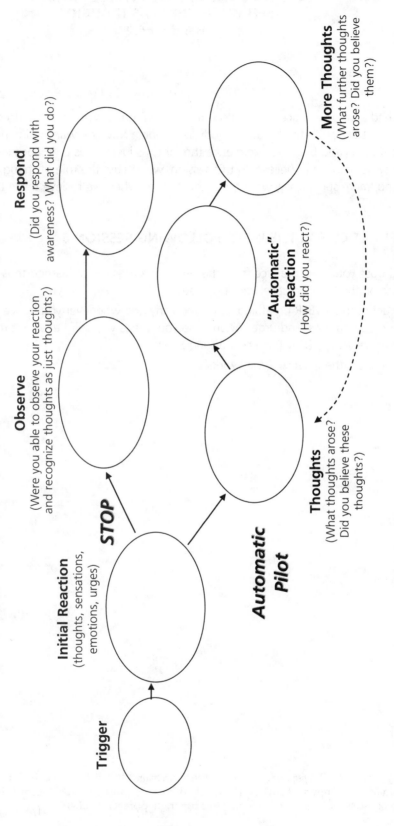

Trigger

Initial Reaction
(thoughts, sensations, emotions, urges)

STOP

Automatic Pilot

Observe
(Were you able to observe your reaction and recognize thoughts as just thoughts?)

Respond
(Did you respond with awareness? What did you do?)

Thoughts
(What thoughts arose? Did you believe these thoughts?)

"Automatic" Reaction
(How did you react?)

More Thoughts
(What further thoughts arose? Did you believe them?)

THEME

We have had a lot of practice noticing our minds wandering. We have practiced gently returning the focus of attention to the breath or body sensations. Now we want to intentionally turn our focus to thoughts and begin to experience thoughts as just words or images in the mind that we may or may not choose to believe. In this session, we discuss the role of thoughts in the relapse process and, more specifically, what tends to happens when we believe these thoughts.

HOME PRACTICE FOR THE WEEK FOLLOWING SESSION 6

1. Choose your own practice from the set of practices we've learned thus far. Note your practice on the Daily Practice Tracking Sheet.
2. Practice the SOBER breathing space regularly and whenever you notice challenging emotions, sensations, and urges or anytime you notice yourself becoming reactive. Note your practice on the Daily Practice Tracking Sheet.
3. Complete the Relapse Cycle Worksheet.

Instructions: Each day, record your meditation practice, also noting any barriers, observations, or comments.

Day/ date	Formal practice with CD: How long?	SOBER breathing space	Notes/comments
	_____ minutes	How many times? In what situations?	
	_____ minutes	How many times? In what situations?	
	_____ minutes	How many times? In what situations?	
	_____ minutes	How many times? In what situations?	
	_____ minutes	How many times? In what situations?	
	_____ minutes	How many times? In what situations?	
	_____ minutes	How many times? In what situations?	

SESSION 7

Self-Care and Lifestyle Balance

Compassion is like a circle that is only complete when
it holds ourselves. Otherwise it isn't wise compassion;
it doesn't recognize our interconnectedness.
—JACK KORNFIELD

MATERIALS

◆ Bell

◆ Whiteboard/markers

◆ Handout 7.1: Daily Activities Worksheet

◆ Handout 7.2: Reminder Card

◆ Handout 7.3: Session 7 Theme and Home Practice: Self-Care and Lifestyle Balance

◆ Handout 7.4: Daily Practice Tracking Sheet

THEME

We have spent several weeks paying close attention to the specific situations, thoughts, and emotions that put us at risk for relapse. In this session, we take a look at the broader picture of our lives, and identify those aspects that support a healthier, more vital life and those that put us at greater risk. Taking care of oneself and engaging in nourishing activities are an essential part of recovery.

GOALS

◆ Discuss the importance of lifestyle balance and taking care of oneself in reducing vulnerability to relapse.

◆ Discuss the use of regular mindfulness practice as a means of maintaining balance.

◆ Prepare for future high-risk situations using the Reminder Card.

SESSION OUTLINE

◆ Check-In

◆ Sitting Meditation: Lovingkindness (Practice 7.1)

◆ Practice Review

◆ Daily Activities Worksheet

◆ Where Does Relapse Begin?

◆ SOBER Breathing Space

◆ Reminder Cards

◆ Home Practice

◆ Closing

CHECK-IN

In these final sessions, it is useful to begin with a reflection on what elements of the course participants have found to be most valuable and what they intend to continue practicing in their daily lives. The check-in in this session can provide an opportunity for participants to recall and recommit to this intention.

SITTING MEDITATION: LOVINGKINDNESS

In this session, a sitting meditation that focuses on lovingkindness—friendliness, good will, or compassion—is introduced (Practice 7.1). There are several ways to practice lovingkindness and they each typically involve sending well-wishes to self and others, beginning with a beloved friend or benefactor. Traditionally, lovingkindness practice involves bringing attention to a set of well-wishes such as *May I be safe and free from harm. May I be peaceful. May I live with ease.* Individuals may modify these well-wishes as needed and use tools such as visualization. We encourage facilitators to explore these practices in their groups if it feels comfortable and appropriate and to be creative in choosing instructions that seem most genuine and relevant for them.

Practicing lovingkindness often gives rise to feelings of resistance, aversion, or other challenging experiences. Participants may comment that it "didn't work," alluding to a failure to feel kindness toward themselves or others. However, as with all the practices thus far, observing these reactions and difficulties with a kind, nonjudgmental attitude is as much a part of the practice as feelings of well-being, openness, and ease. We have found it useful to address this and remind participants that there is no "right" experience. Lovingkindness practice is not intended to bring about a certain feeling or mind state but rather involves observing whatever arises as we practice.

PRACTICE REVIEW

Over the previous week, participants have been engaging in their own patterns of practice. As part of the practice review, we invite participants to share what they are noticing in the process of making the practice "their own," whether they have been able to find a routine that feels sustainable, and address ongoing barriers and challenges. Participants have also been continuing their practice of the SOBER space and may have experiences to share. Finally, they were asked to complete the Relapse Cycle Worksheet (Handout 6.1), using an example that was relevant for them. Sharing a few examples helps reiterate the importance of "stepping out" of the relapse process as early as possible and sets the stage for Session 7, in which we widen our focus to a broader picture of relapse risks and lifestyle balance.

DAILY ACTIVITIES WORKSHEET

The Daily Activities Worksheet (Handout 7.1), an adaptation of exercises from MBCT (Segal et al., 2002) and from Daley and Marlatt's (2006) relapse prevention protocol, is a tool intended to bring awareness to typical daily activities and how they tend to affect overall mood, life balance, and health, discussed in terms of "nourishing" and "depleting" effects. This daily activities exercise encourages reflection on the manner in which we engage in these activities and whether there are ways we tend to make a "neutral" activity depleting or a neutral or depleting activity more nourishing. It is an opportunity to have participants notice the actual qualities of each experience and to differentiate those from additional "layers" they may be adding that make it more depleting.

In Part 1 of this exercise, using the Daily Activities Worksheet participants compile lists of activities, people, and situations in their lives that feel depleting (e.g., discouraging, exhausting, frustrating, draining) and that feel nourishing (e.g., energizing, pleasurable, rejuvenating, satisfying). Participants then describe how they tend to feel during or after the activity. In Part 2 of this exercise, participants list on the back of the worksheet activities of a typical day and then review the list and identify each activity as either nourishing ("N") or depleting ("D"). Participants then tally the "Ns" and the "Ds."

Participants are often surprised by having either more nourishing activities or more depleting activities in their day than they anticipated. They often remark on how the same activity may be nourishing or depleting depending on their state of mind, other factors in their lives, or the way in which they approach it. This exercise not only offers perspective on how we spend our days and the balance between depleting versus nourishing activities, but also elicits discussion of the importance of including more nourishing activities or engaging in activities in a way that might be less depleting.

The purpose of this exercise is not to encourage them to eradicate all depleting activities (although the addition of more daily activities that feed us in a healthful way, even seemingly small ones, certainly has benefits to our mood and functioning). Rather, it is intended to begin to bring greater awareness to how we spend our days, the quality of attention and presence we bring to our activities, and how both the activities and our quality of attention to them tend to affect us. Some depleting or stressful activities might be avoidable; others are not. This is an opportunity for us to notice what is nourishing and depleting and to explore how we might relate to experiences differently. Further, discussion can also include how mindfulness practice helps this process and how the ways we relate to daily activities might invite relapse.

Home practice for this session includes choosing at least three activities that are nourishing and engaging in them over the upcoming week. It is important that participants choose activities that are realistic and that they can commit to. These can either be new activities or ones in which they already engage. It can be helpful to have participants state aloud what activities they are committing to.

WHERE DOES RELAPSE BEGIN?

Until now, discussions and exercises have focused largely on the acute triggers for relapse (e.g., people, places, thoughts, emotions). This session begins to widen the focus to lifestyle choices that make us more or less vulnerable to relapse.

For example, imagine that a participant is walking down a street and sees someone with whom she used to drink. On a particular day, she may be able to handle this situation skillfully, choosing to turn the corner and take a different route or to say hello, tell her friend she is no longer drinking, and continue walking. On another day, she might encounter this same friend and choose to engage in conversation, not mention to her friend that she is in recovery, accept the friend's invitation to go to their favorite bar to see some old friends, and then end up with a drink. In reviewing factors that may affect one's vulnerability in this situation, we elicit examples from the group, such as general stress level, exhaustion, loneliness, and lack of social support. We often mention the acronym HALT (*H*ungry, *A*ngry, *L*onely, *T*ired) from the 12-step tradition as examples of factors influencing vulnerability. In this exercise, it is helpful to highlight that these are common experiences that will continue to arise in our lives. Recognizing them as warning signs can remind us to take better care of ourselves and alert us to our increased vulnerability to triggers during these times. It can be helpful to check in when feeling triggered ("Am I hungry? Sad? Lonely? Anxious?") as a way to understand our reaction to a trigger and to identify what we need to do to best take care of ourselves ("What is it I really need right now?").

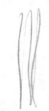

SOBER BREATHING SPACE

Often after discussions, especially those that can become abstract or conceptual, facilitators might suggest pausing with a SOBER breathing space. It can be helpful to practice these in different ways throughout the course. For example, facilitators might suggest trying the exercise with eyes open and might vary the length of time spent engaged in the exercise. These variations can help increase flexibility and generalizability of this practice.

REMINDER CARDS

The Reminder Card (Handout 7.2) is intended as a constant resource for support. About the size of a business card, it contains four sections (two on each side) of support information: participants' personalized list of reasons for continuing to choose sobriety, most effective alternative coping behaviors, emergency or support telephone numbers, and the steps of the SOBER breathing space. The Reminder Card is easily carried in a pocket or wallet, readily accessible for general reminding and for use in high-risk situations.

Certain individuals, particularly those who are relatively early in their recovery and who are seeking concrete tools and reminders, may find the Reminder Card to be helpful. Others (e.g., individuals who have been in recovery for a longer period of time), however, may not find it as relevant. Thus, we encourage facilitators to consider this as optional, depending on the specific needs of the group. Ideally, the Reminder Card is discussed and completed in session because participants can benefit from others' thoughts and ideas. For example, some participants might share a significant reason for maintaining sobriety that is particularly powerful or salient for another and thus important to include on the card.

In generating effective coping behaviors, it can be helpful to invite participants to take a moment to think first about the elements that place them at high risk for relapse; these can be people, places, situations, thoughts, or emotions. From there, they can identify the specific steps they can take to help them cope. Following this, we briefly review the steps of the SOBER practice noted on the card.

The final quadrant of the Reminder Card contains phone numbers of local community resources and help lines, and participants are instructed to supplement this with contact information for their own personal resources or support systems. The Reminder Card should be completed with this additional information before the next session.

HOME PRACTICE

For the upcoming week, we continue to encourage group members to create their own practice routine, choosing a practice they intend to use on a regular basis and engaging in it for 6 out of the next 7 days. We also suggest continued practice of the SOBER breathing space, both during routine daily activities and in higher stress situations. Finally, we review the plan to engage in three specific nourishing activities (Handout 7.3), and instruct participants to complete the Reminder Card if there are additional ideas or resources they would like to add. Participants are also instructed to record meditation practice on the Daily Practice Tracking Sheet (Handout 7.4).

CLOSING

The last few moments of the session can provide another opportunity to have participants recall and reconnect with their practice intentions that they identified at the beginning of the session.

This meditation is slightly different from those we have practiced in the course thus far. It is a "friendliness" or compassion practice that involves developing a kinder, gentler attitude toward ourselves and others. This compassionate and friendly approach is an important aspect of mindfulness practice and can help support the other practices that we have done.

To begin, find a position that is comfortable for you, allowing your body to be completely at ease and beginning by just loosening any tension in your body. Allowing any tightness in your body to release, softening your belly, gently releasing any tension in your arms and shoulders, your face, relaxing your jaw. Maybe taking a moment to connect with your intention, your reason for being here and engaging in this practice.

Feeling your body against the floor or the chair. Feeling the solidity and stability of the ground beneath you, allowing your body to release into the chair or the ground, and feeling a sense of safety here in this moment, allowing the ground to support you.

Now bring to mind someone you know personally, or know of, who is easy to love and toward whom you naturally have feelings of friendliness and caring. This may be a friend, a child, a grandchild or grandparent. Or it could be a spiritual guide, or even a pet. It is best not to pick someone with whom you've had conflict or to whom you are romantically involved, but rather just someone toward whom you feel an easy warmth and friendliness. Maybe someone who makes you naturally smile just by thinking about him or her.

If you'd like, imagine that this someone is sitting next to you, by your side, or in front of you. If you are unable to picture this person, just allow yourself to focus on the feeling, the sensations you may experience in the presence of this being. Take a few minutes to pay attention to how you feel, sensing where in your body you experience feelings of compassion and caring. This may be in the center of your chest, where your heart is, or in the belly or the face. Wherever you feel the experience of caring or kindness in your body, with each breath, allow this area to soften. If you have trouble sensing this or finding the area where these feelings might be centered, it's okay. Just keep your focus on this general area of your heart and notice what, if anything, you can sense there throughout this exercise.

Now, if it feels comfortable to you, send this being well-wishes. We often use the following, repeating them quietly in our minds:

> *May you be safe and protected. May you find true happiness. May you be peaceful. May you live with ease.* (Repeat slowly.)

You can use these well-wishes or you can create your own, whatever feels most genuine for you. Continuing to repeat them mentally. *May you be safe and protected. May you be happy. May you be peaceful. May you live with ease.* Or whatever well-wishes you have chosen.

(cont.)

The idea is not to make anything happen; we are simply sending well-wishes, the way you might wish someone a safe journey or a good day. If you find yourself having thoughts such as, "This isn't working" or "This is silly," just noticing these thoughts and gently guiding your attention back to the wishes. Similarly, if you find yourself feeling frustrated or irritated, just bringing your attention to that experience, and remembering that you can always bring your attention back to simply sensing the area where your heart is. Reminding yourself that there is nothing in particular that you are supposed to feel when you do this practice. Just allowing your experience to be your experience.

Now imagine that this person is sending the same well-wishes to you. *May you be safe and protected. May you be happy. May you be peaceful. May you live with ease.*

If it feels comfortable, you may shift your attention now from this person to yourself and send yourself the well-wishes—*May I be safe and protected. May I be happy. May I be peaceful. May I live with ease*—or whatever wishes you have chosen. And with each wish taking a moment to feel that wish in your body and heart. What does "safe" feel like? How does "happy" feel? So that you are able to connecting with these wishes.

If it is easier, you may imagine yourself as a young child receiving these well-wishes. If you find yourself having judging thoughts or thinking *about* the exercise, just noticing these thoughts and guiding your attention back to the phrases. If you notice any resistance or anxiety, as best you can, allowing that resistance to soften. Seeing if you can have compassion for your experience, just as it is. Continuing to experiment with this on your own for a few more minutes.

Now sending these wishes to the people in the room with you. *May we be safe and protected. May we be happy. May we be peaceful. May we live with ease.* Again, using whatever wishes feel most comfortable and meaningful to you. There is no need to force any particular feeling here—just simply extending wishes to yourself and the others here with you.

Take a moment to receive these wishes that the others in the room have sent to you.

Whenever you are ready, you may allow your eyes to open.

DAILY ACTIVITIES WORKSHEET
Handout 7.1

1. List activities, people and situations that you associate with **distress, and challenging emotions** or that increase **self-doubt,** and describe how you tend to feel when you engage in these activities.

   Activity, person, place, or situation   How do you tend to feel?

   _____   _____

   _____   _____

   _____   _____

   _____   _____

   _____   _____

2. List activities, people, and situations that you associate with **pleasure** or that increase your **confidence** that don't involve substance use. Note how you tend to feel when engaged in these activities.

   Activity, person, place, or situation   How do you tend to feel?

   _____   _____

   _____   _____

   _____   _____

   _____   _____

Side One | Side Two

REASONS TO STAY SOBER

-
-
-
-
-

CONTACT NUMBERS

-
-
-
-
-

- SOBER BREATHING SPACE
- Stop: pause wherever you are
- Observe: notice what's going on right now
- Breathe: direct focus to your breathing
- Expand your awareness
- Respond with awareness

ALTERNATE ACTIVITIES/PLANS

-
-
-
-
-

THEME

We have spent several weeks paying close attention to the specific situations, thoughts, and emotions that put us at risk for relapse. Taking care of ourselves and engaging in nourishing activities are also crucial parts of recovery. In this session, we take a look at the broader picture of our lives and identify aspects that support a healthier, more vital life as well as those that put us at risk. Lifestyle balance and compassion for oneself can be essential elements of a healthy and fulfilling life.

HOME PRACTICE FOR THE WEEK FOLLOWING SESSION 7

1. Among all the different forms of practice, choose a pattern you intend to use on a regular basis (e.g., sitting three times per week and body scan three times per week or simply sitting six times per week). Engage in your chosen program this week.

2. Practice the SOBER breathing space three or more times a day (regular times and whenever you notice unpleasant thoughts, feelings, or cravings).

3. Engage in at least three nourishing activities that you have marked on your Daily Activities Worksheet.

4. Finish filling out the reminder card, if you haven't already done so.

DAILY PRACTICE TRACKING SHEET
Handout 7.4

Instructions: Each day, record your meditation practice, also noting any barriers, observations, or comments.

Day/ date	Formal practice with CD: How long?	SOBER breathing space	Notes/comments
	_____ minutes	How many times? In what situations?	
	_____ minutes	How many times? In what situations?	
	_____ minutes	How many times? In what situations?	
	_____ minutes	How many times? In what situations?	
	_____ minutes	How many times? In what situations?	
	_____ minutes	How many times? In what situations?	
	_____ minutes	How many times? In what situations?	

Social Support and Continuing Practice

This road demands courage and stamina, yet it's full of footprints.
Who are these companions?
They are rungs in your ladder. Use them!
With company you quicken your ascent.
You'll be happy enough going along, but with others, you'll get farther, and faster.

—RUMI

MATERIALS

◆ Bell

◆ Whiteboard/markers

◆ Pebbles

◆ Handout 8.1: Resource List

◆ Handout 8.2: Reflections on the Course Worksheet

◆ Handout 8.3: Session 8 Theme: Social Support and Continuing Practice

THEME

Recovery and mindfulness practice are both lifelong journeys that require commitment and diligence. This is not an easy voyage. In fact, it can feel at times like swimming upstream. Thus far, we have learned about factors that put us at risk, some skills to help navigate through high-risk situations, and about the importance of maintaining lifestyle balance. Hopefully participating in this group has also provided a sense of support and community. Having a support network is crucial to continuing along the path of practice and recovery. Having a recovery support system can help us recognize signs of relapse and provide support when we feel we are at risk. Having support around our meditation practice can help us sustain our practice and choose to show up for our lives in a mindful, intentional, and compassionate way.

GOALS

◆ Highlight the importance of support networks as a way of reducing risk and maintaining recovery.

◆ Find ways to overcome barriers to asking for help.

◆ Reflect on what participants have learned from the course and reasons for continuing practice.

◆ Develop a plan for continued practice and incorporation of mindfulness in daily life.

SESSION OUTLINE

◆ Check-In

◆ Body Scan (Practice 8.1)

◆ Practice Review

◆ The Importance of Support Networks

◆ Reflections on the Course

◆ Intentions for the Future

◆ Concluding Meditation (Practice 8.2)

◆ Closing Circle

CHECK-IN

Participants are invited to share one or two words describing a sensation, quality of mind, or emotion they are noticing. Rather than planning what they are going to say, facilitators might encourage them to listen and be present for the other group members as they share their experiences.

BODY SCAN

The body scan was practiced in the very first MBRP session. It can be useful to revisit this, giving participants a marker by which to assess changes that might have occurred over the past 2 months. Facilitators might ask about the experience of the practice and what has changed and what has stayed the same since the beginning of the course. We have sometimes shared the poem "The Paradox" at the end of this session's body scan meditation (Practice 8.1).

PRACTICE REVIEW

Practice review includes the previous week's meditation practice and a check-in on the process of establishing an individualized sustainable practice. We also review experiences with the SOBER breathing space, review completion and use of the Reminder Card (Handout 7.2), and discuss the nourishing activities home practice exercise (as described in Handout 7.3). The facilitator can ask about what participants noticed when doing these activities, the quality of experience of engaging in the nourishing activities, and how we can bring some of those qualities into activities that feel more depleting. It is useful to reflect on how mindfulness practice can change the quality of and relationship to activities. Equally important as reviewing participants' experiences of engaging in these activities is helping them to identify barriers to engaging in nourishing activities.

THE IMPORTANCE OF SUPPORT NETWORKS

The previous sessions have explored several strategies, practices, and skills for coping with stressful or risky situations. The focus then widened to consider broader lifestyle choices and how those may be contributing to or detracting from our intended direction. Here we expand the lens further, to look at our communities and environments (Handout 8.3).

Asking participants why support is important may seem an obvious question. It may help them to recognize, however, how crucial a system of support is to both recovery and sustaining a regular mindfulness practice. Neither of these paths is meant to be traveled alone; we need companions. We need encouragement and reminders to continue on this challenging journey. We often have participants offer their ideas and experiences of ways to find and maintain support for both recovery and mindfulness practice. Identifying possible barriers ahead of time can be useful in recognizing and working with them if and when they arise, so we often ask participants to anticipate what might get in the way of asking for help or maintaining a support network. We typically also review current resources, such as family, friends, and 12-step or other support groups.

Finally, we offer a list of meditation resources (Handout 8.1), which can include not only websites, books, and CDs but also local meetings, courses, and retreats.

If feasible, ongoing meditation practice sessions as part of the MBRP program can be offered, providing a safe and familiar venue to support participants' ongoing practice.

REFLECTIONS ON THE COURSE

In this final session of the course, we give participants an opportunity to reflect, individually and as a group, on their experiences over the past 2 months. We also invite them to look ahead and create an intention for continued practice. The Reflections on the Course Worksheet (Handout 8.2) asks about experiences of being in the course and gives participants an opportunity to provide feedback or suggestions for changes to the content and structure. We typically allow 10 minutes for worksheet completion, and remind the group that their feedback is highly valued, will remain anonymous, and will be used for the improvement of future courses.

Before collecting these sheets, we invite participants to share anything they wrote or any other reflections they might have from the course. Participants typically welcome and appreciate this opportunity to share any final thoughts, comments, or questions with the group.

INTENTIONS FOR THE FUTURE

Allowing participants to identify the importance of continued practice can be much more powerful than having facilitators preach the merits of daily meditation. We begin this exercise by asking the participants why they might maintain this practice, compiling their ideas and writing them on the whiteboard. We often follow this by asking participants to state individually what type of practice they intend to carry forward and how likely they are to continue with practice.

> FACILITATOR: It will be up to each of you to decide if and how you integrate and continue mindfulness practice in your lives. If you do continue, what are some ways the practice might be helpful or important in your life?
>
> PARTICIPANT 1: I used to make things more rigid or complicated than they needed to be, and I still do, but I can catch myself on occasion—my mind going there. This helps me stay in the here and now and not future trip or obsess about the past and get so stuck there.
>
> PARTICIPANT 2: Keeping my awareness and being alert. Keeping my observation sharp and focused. That can tend to get dull if I don't practice. If I don't work at it, and just allow myself to be unaware, that can lead me back to relapse.

Similar to recognizing risks for relapse and identifying unhelpful patterns before they occur, it can be useful to identify barriers to continuing practice and the beginning signs of "falling off the meditation wagon":

FACILITATOR: Practice often evolves over time, so it is important to commit here to a practice, and also be aware that this is a lifetime pursuit and will go through many changes. What do you anticipate might get in the way?

PARTICIPANT 3: Time.

FACILITATOR: So finding time, setting time aside. That's a big one for people. What else?

PARTICIPANT 4: Laziness.

FACILITATOR: Okay. So what is laziness, really? What is that like or how might that play out?

PARTICIPANT 2: Like before I relapse, I stop going to meetings. I stop associating with clean people. I start doing old behaviors.

FACILITATOR: Disconnecting from the newer behaviors and falling back into old behavior patterns that are pretty familiar.

PARTICIPANT 2: Yeah. I slack on things that I know are good or healthy for me.

FACILITATOR: So what do we do when this stuff gets in the way? This is natural and it will happen. We'll make excuses, and maybe miss a day or two, then have that experience of the abstinence violation effect, like "I knew I couldn't do this." It's important to recognize the possibility—the probability—of this up front and to remember that we can always begin again, any day, in any moment. So if you begin to feel stuck or lose interest or find that your practice is starting to fade, what are some strategies that might help?

PARTICIPANT 2: Set a time, really schedule it into the day.

FACILITATOR: Yes. What else? What about when those excuses or that doubt comes up?

PARTICIPANT 3: Agreeing with myself that no matter what I think or how I feel, I just sit. Doing it first thing in the morning, so I just get up and sit right away without thinking too much about it.

FACILITATOR: So making it easy for yourself. Keeping the cushion or CD out, so it's right there and available. Committing to getting on the cushion, even if it isn't for the whole 30 or 40 minutes. Even if it's just for 2 minutes, just staying in the habit.

PARTICIPANT 1: Yeah, otherwise I get hard on myself, and it feels too big—"Oh, I can't do 45 minutes."

FACILITATOR: So even if this does happen, say a month passes and it feels way too far away, you can always begin again. You haven't "lost" it. There's no need to waste your time judging yourself. Just start again at the beginning. Always, always remembering that this practice is about compassion and about being kind to yourself. This is not another thing to beat yourself up over; it's the very opposite. This is a way to really take care of yourself, unconditionally and with a very whole and gentle compassion.

CONCLUDING MEDITATION

The concluding meditation (Practice 8.2) honors each person's journey over the past 2 months, and offers a brief metta or lovingkindness meditation for self, fellow participants, friends and family, and finally all sentient beings. We invite each person to choose a small stone from a collection we bring to the final group as a symbol of the rough, natural, flawed-yet-perfect beauty of each human being. It is reminder of this journey that participants can take with them, to carry in a pocket, or place on a desk, bedside table, or mantel.

CLOSING CIRCLE

We close the final session of the course by sitting in a circle, opening up the last moments for any final thoughts or reflections. Participants are welcome to share any final comments but are also welcome to just sit quietly. As with each of the prior sessions, the final moments are in silence, closing the session with the sound of the bell.

BODY SCAN
Practice 8.1

The body scan practice from Session 1 is repeated. We close the practice in this final session with a poem.

A poem by Gunilla Norris:*

PARADOX

It is a paradox that we encounter so much internal noise
when we first try to sit in silence.

It is a paradox that experiencing pain releases pain.

It is a paradox that keeping still can lead us
so fully into life and being.

Our minds do not like paradoxes. We want things
to be clear, so we can maintain our illusions of safety.
Certainty breeds tremendous smugness.

We each possess a deeper level of being, however,
which loves paradox. It knows that summer is already
growing like a seed in the depth of winter. It knows
that the moment we are born, we begin to die. It knows
that all of life shimmers, in shades of becoming—
that shadow and light are always together,
the visible mingled with the invisible.

When we sit in stillness we are profoundly active.
Keeping silent, we can hear the roar of existence.
Through our willingness to be the one we are,
we become one with everything.

Now very slowly and gently, while still maintaining an awareness of your body, when you are ready, open your eyes and allow your awareness to include the room and the rest of the people here.

---

*From *Sharing Silence: Meditation Practice and Mindful Living* by Gunilla Norris. Copyright 1992 by Gunilla Norris. Used by permission of Harmony Books, a division of Random House, Inc.

CONCLUDING MEDITATION
Practice 8.2

I am going to go around with this bowl of stones. Please pick one that you are drawn to or that speaks to you. As best you can, bringing all of your attention to this object, just like you did on the very first day of this course, holding it in the palm of your hand. Examining it as though you had never seen anything like it before.

Taking a moment to turn it over, observing its color and texture, noticing places where the light hits it, noticing the sensation of it in your hand. If any thoughts come to you while you are doing this, then just noting them as thoughts and bringing your attention back to the object. Perhaps reflect on the richness of its history—the thousands of years, the weather, the force of gravity—that formed this object. Noticing that it isn't perfectly round, that it may have cracks and crevices, but that we wouldn't say it is imperfect.

Allowing this object to be a reminder for you, of having been in this course, of everything that you experienced and all of the energy and hard work you have put into this practice. And knowing that you too have a rich history that has shaped you, that you may not be perfectly shaped. Maybe you have your own cracks and crevices.

You may take a moment to close your eyes, while continuing to feel this object. Maybe closing your hand around the object. Taking a few moments to appreciate yourself, all the effort it took to be here and engage in this group and these practices and your commitment to your recovery. Appreciate, too, the commitment of all the others who have shared this experience with you.

Above all, let this object be a reminder of your journey, everything that has brought you to this point in your recovery, and of continuing the process that you have started, discovering a way of being present and living alongside all the aspects of yourself, including those that may seem damaged or imperfect. Responding to them and holding them with gentleness and caring attention.

Taking a moment now to wish yourself well. If you'd like, you may focus on the well-wishes that we practiced with in the previous session and repeat them to yourself quietly, holding the stone in your hand—*May I be safe. May I be happy. May I be peaceful. May I live with ease*—or any other wishes that feel genuine and natural for you.

Just continuing to repeat them a few times, taking them in with each breath, and allowing yourself to find a sense of caring and tenderness for yourself as you do this. And if you find your mind wandering or notice other thoughts coming up, just noticing them, without judgment, and guiding your attention back to the well-wishes.

And then taking a moment to think of the person sitting to the right of you, of everything that has brought them to this point in their lives, of the struggles that they may have experienced along the way, and of how, like you, they are working hard to continue along this path and maintain their recovery. So taking a moment to wish them well on their journey and send your caring wishes to them. *May you be safe. May you be happy. May you be peaceful. May you live with ease.* And thinking of the person to the left of you and wishing him or her well.

(cont.)

Continuing to go around the room in this way, wishing each person well. *May each one of us be safe, happy, peaceful, and live with ease.* Now taking a moment to receive the wishes sent to you from the others here in the group, knowing that everyone here has wished you well.

Sections based on Segal, Williams, and Teasdale (2002).

WEBSITES

- Downloadable meditation teachings and instruction from Dharma Seed: *www.dharmaseed. org*
- Meditation instructions, including mindfulness of breath and lovingkindness or compassion meditation: *www.lisadalemiller.com/meditations.htm*
- Meditation CDs for addiction, relapse prevention, stress, anxiety, and depression: *drsgoldstein.com/CDs.aspx*
- Meditation CDs and tapes developed by Jon Kabat-Zinn for the MBSR program: *www.mindfulnesscds.com/series1.html*
- Teachings, discussions, resources, listings of retreats: *www.dharmapunx.com*
- Links and articles relevant to meditation and recovery: *www.buddhistrecovery.org*

BOOKS

- *Dharma Punx: A Memoir,* by Noah Levine. New York: Harper San Francisco, 2003.
- *Insight Meditation: The Practice of Freedom,* by Joseph Goldstein. Boston: Shambhala, 1993.
- *The Mindful Path to Self-Compassion: Freeing Yourself from Destructive Thoughts and Emotions,* by Christopher K. Germer. New York: Guilford Press, 2009.
- *Mindful Recovery: A Spiritual Path to Healing from Addiction,* by Thomas Bien and Beverly Bien. New York: Wiley, 2002.
- *The Mindful Way through Anxiety: Break Free from Chronic Worry and Reclaim Your Life,* by Susan M. Orsillo and Lizabeth Roemer. New York: Guilford Press, 2011.
- *The Mindful Way through Depression: Freeing Yourself from Chronic Unhappiness,* by J. Mark G. Williams, John D. Teasdale, Zindel V. Segal, and Jon Kabat-Zinn. New York: Guilford Press, 2007.
- *The Mindfulness Solution: Everyday Practices for Everyday Problems,* by Ronald D. Siegel. New York: Guilford Press, 2010.
- *The Miracle of Mindfulness: An Introduction to the Practice of Meditation,* by Thich Nhat Hanh. Boston: Beacon Press, 1987.
- *One Breath at a Time: Buddhism and the Twelve Steps,* by Kevin Griffin. Emmaus, PA: Rodale, 2004.

(cont.)

- *A Path with Heart: A Guide through the Perils and Promises of Spiritual Life,* by Jack Kornfield. New York: Bantam, 1993.
- *Radical Acceptance: Embracing Your Life with the Heart of a Buddha,* by Tara Brach. New York: Bantam, 2003.
- *Seeking the Heart of Wisdom: The Path of Insight Meditation,* by Joseph Goldstein and Jack Kornfield. Boston: Shambhala, 1987.
- *Start Where You Are: A Guide to Compassionate Living,* by Pema Chödrön. Boston: Shambhala, 1994.
- *When Things Fall Apart: Heart Advice for Difficult Times,* by Pema Chödrön, Boston: Shambhala, 1997.
- *Wherever You Go, There You Are: Mindfulness Meditation in Everyday Life,* by Jon Kabat-Zinn. New York: Hyperion, 1994.

Please take a moment to reflect upon the following questions and write down your responses:

1. What did you find most valuable about this course? What, if anything, did you learn?

2. What, if anything, has changed for you over the past 8 weeks as a result of your participation?

3. Was there anything that got in the way of your learning or growth or that might have improved the course for you?

4. Other comments?

5. On a scale of 1 (*not at all*) to 10 (*very*), how important has this program been to you? Please explain why you have given it this rating.

6. On a scale of 1 (*not at all*) to 10 (*very*), how likely are you to continue engaging in **formal** mindfulness practice (e.g., body scan, sitting meditation, mindful stretching/yoga) after this course?

7. On a scale of 1 (*not at all*) to 10 (*very*), how likely are you to continue engaging in **informal** mindfulness practice (e.g., SOBER breathing space, mindful eating, walking, daily activities) after this course?

Using the mindfulness skills we've learned over the past 8 weeks can help us face our experiences differently; we can accept the experience instead of fighting it, and from there make choices that are coming from a wiser, more spacious place. This moment-by-moment journey of recovery and mindfulness practice can feel, at times, like swimming upstream. It is not an easy voyage. Thus far, we have learned about the factors that put us at risk, some skills to help navigate through high-risk situations, and the importance of maintaining lifestyle balance.

Participating in this group has also hopefully provided a sense of support and community. Having a support network is crucial to continuing along the path of practice and recovery. Having a recovery support system can help us recognize signs of relapse and provide encouragement when we feel we are at risk. Having support around our meditation practice can help us maintain our practice and choose to show up for our lives.

There are many things we do not have control over and many things that may not go "our way." We do have a choice, however, in how we respond and how we experience our lives. Practicing mindfulness on a regular basis helps us be less automatic and reactive and more aware in our choices, ultimately giving us greater freedom. Taking care of ourselves and engaging in activities that nourish us is part of maintaining balance in our lives and helping protect against relapse. Maintaining a practice is not easy. Difficulties and barriers will arise. Be gentle with yourself. Remember that any practice is good practice; you can always begin again from right where you are.

References

Barks, C. (Trans.). (1995). *The essential Rumi*. San Francisco: Harper.

Benson, M. D. H. (1975). *The relaxation response*. New York: William Morrow.

Bowen, S., Chawla, N., Collins, S., Witkiewitz, K., Hsu, S., Grow, J., Clifasefi, S., Garner, M., Douglass, A., Larimer, M., & Marlatt, G. A. (2009). Mindfulness-based relapse prevention for substance use disorders: A pilot efficacy trial. *Substance Abuse, 30*, 205–305.

Bowen, S., Witkiewitz, K., Dillworth, T., Chawla, N., Simpson, T., Ostafin, B., Larimer, M. E., Blume, A., Parks, G., & Marlatt, G. A. (2006). Mindfulness meditation and substance use in an incarcerated population. *Psychology of Addictive Behaviors, 20*, 343–347.

Brewer, J., Sinha, R., Chen, J. A., Michalsen, R. N., Babuscio, T. A., Nich, C., Grier, A., Bergquist, K. L., Reis, A. L., Potenza, M. N., Carroll, K. M., & Rounsaville, B. J. (2009). Mindfulness training and stress reactivity in substance abuse: Results from a randomized, controlled stage I pilot study. *Substance Abuse, 30*, 306–317.

Curry, S., Marlatt, G. A., & Gordon, J. R. (1987). Abstinence violation effect: Validation of an attributional construct with smoking cessation. *Journal of Consulting and Clinical Psychology, 55*, 145–149.

Daley, D., & Marlatt, G.A. (2006). *Overcoming your drug or alcohol problem: Effective recovery strategies*. New York: Oxford University Press.

Donnenfield, D. (Producer/director). (1998). *Changing from inside* [DVD]. Onalaska, WA: Pariyatti.

Frankl, V. E. (1946). *Man's search for meaning*. Boston: Beacon Press.

Griffin, K. (2004). *One breath at a time: Buddhism and the twelve steps*. Emmaus, PA: Rodale.

Kabat-Zinn, J. (1990). *Full catastrophe living: Using the wisdom of your body and mind to face stress, pain, and illness*. New York: Delacorte.

Kabat-Zinn, J. (1994). *Wherever you go, there you are: Mindfulness meditation in everyday life*. New York: Hyperion.

Kabat-Zinn, J. (2002). *Guided mindfulness meditation* [CD recording]. Lexington, MA: Sounds True, Inc.

Kabat-Zinn, J. (2003). Mindfulness-based interventions in context: Past, present, and future. *Clinical Psychology Science and Practice, 10*, 144–156.

Kabat-Zinn, J., Massion, A., Kristeller, J., Peterson, L. G., Fletcher, K. E., Pbert, L., Lenderking, W. R., & Santorelli, S. F. (1992). Effectiveness of a meditation-based stress reduction intervention in the treatment of anxiety disorders. *American Journal of Psychiatry, 149,* 936–943.

Kornfield, J. (2004). *A path with heart* [CD recording]. Lexington, MA: Sounds True, Inc.

Marlatt, G. A., & Donovan, P. M. (Eds.). (2005). *Relapse prevention: Maintenance strategies in the treatment of addictive behaviors* (2nd ed.). New York: Guilford Press.

Marlatt, G. A. (2002). Buddhist philosophy and the treatment of addictive behavior. *Cognitive and Behavioral Practice, 9,* 44–50.

Marlatt, G. A., & Gordon, J. R. (Eds.). (1985). *Relapse prevention: Maintenance strategies in the treatment of addictive behaviors.* New York: Guilford Press.

Marlatt, G. A., & Marques, J. K. (1977). Meditation, self-control, and alcohol use. In R. B. Stuart (Ed.), *Behavioral self-management: Strategies, techniques, and outcomes* (pp. 117–153). New York: Brunner/Mazel.

Marlatt, G. A., Pagano, R. R., Rose, R. M., & Marques, J. K. (1984). Effects of meditation and relaxation training upon alcohol use in male social drinkers. In D. H. Shapiro & R. N. Walsh (Eds.), *Meditation: Classic and contemporary perspectives*(pp. 105–120). New York: Aldine.

Marlatt, G. A., & Witkiewitz, K. (2005). Relapse prevention for alcohol and drug problems. In G. A. Marlatt & D. M. Donovan (Eds.), *Relapse prevention: Maintenance strategies in the treatment of addictive behaviors* (2nd ed., pp. 1–44). New York: Guilford Press.

Moyers, B. (1993). *Healing and the mind: Vol. 3. Healing from within* [Video recording]. New York: Public Broadcasting Service.

Norris, G. (1992). *Sharing silence: Meditation practice and mindful living.* New York: Harmony Books.

Okulitch, P. V., & Marlatt, G. A. (1972). The effects of varied extinction conditions with alcoholics and social drinkers. *Journal of Abnormal Psychology, 79,* 205–211.

Roth, B., & Creasor, T. (1997). Mindfulness meditation-based stress reduction: Experience with a bilingual inner-city program. *Nurse Practitioner, 22,* 150–176.

Santorelli, S. (1998). *Heal thyself: Lessons on mindfulness and medicine.* New York: Random House.

Segal, Z. V., Williams, J. M. G., & Teasdale, J. D. (2002). *Mindfulness-based cognitive therapy for depression.* New York: Guilford Press.

Spicer, J. (1993). *The Minnesota model: The evolution of the multidisciplinary approach to addiction recovery.* Center City, MN: Hazelden.

Teasdale, J. D., Segal, Z. V., Williams, J. M. G., Ridgeway, V. A., Soulsby, J. M., & Lau, M. A., (2000). Prevention of relapse/recurrence in major depression by mindfulness-based cognitive therapy. *Journal of Consulting and Clinical Psychology, 68,* 615–623.

Witkiewitz, K., Marlatt, G. A., & Walker, D. (2005). Mindfulness-based relapse prevention for alcohol and substance use disorders. *Journal of Cognitive Psychotherapy, 19,* 211–228.

Zgierska, A., Rabago, D., Zuelsdorff, M., Coe, C., Miller, M., & Fleming, M. (2008). Mindfulness meditation for alcohol relapse prevention: A feasibility pilot study. *Journal of Addiction Medicine, 2,* 165–173.

Index